...moved to London from Colorado in 1989 seeking a career as a theatre director, but swiftly developed a passion for cooking and changed tack. She forged a career as a chef, food writer and businesswoman. Starting as a private chef for film director Stanley Kubrick and family, she went on to author several cookbooks.

Celia created her highly successful food tour business, Gastrotours, in 2002, as a platform to share her passion. She connects people with an array of artisan foods around London's gastronomic hotspots, including Borough Market and Portobello. Her extensive knowledge, curiosity and constant engagement with markets and ingredients have firmly established her as a top food expert.

She has had eight cookbooks published worldwide and numerous journalistic accomplishments, with columns for *The Times*, *BBC Good Food Magazine* and *The Evening Standard*, and currently writes for the Borough Market blog and the market's resident magazine, *Market Life*. She has also made multiple TV appearances. Her cooking style is fundamentally vegetarian, and she is also known as "The New Urban Farmer", writing about growing to eat, based on her experience tending her London allotment.

Find out more at www.celiabrooksbrown.com

Low-Carb & Gluten-Free
VEGETARIAN

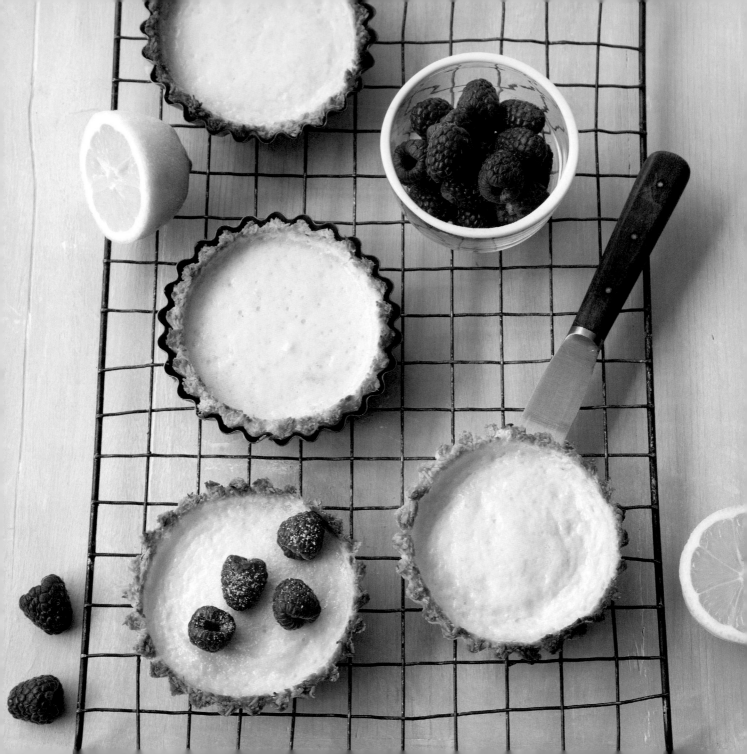

Low-Carb & Gluten-Free
VEGETARIAN

SIMPLE, DELICIOUS RECIPES FOR A LOW-CARB AND GLUTEN-FREE LIFESTYLE

Celia Brooks

Photography by Clare Winfield
Nutritional analysis by Fiona Hunter and Anita Bean

PAVILION

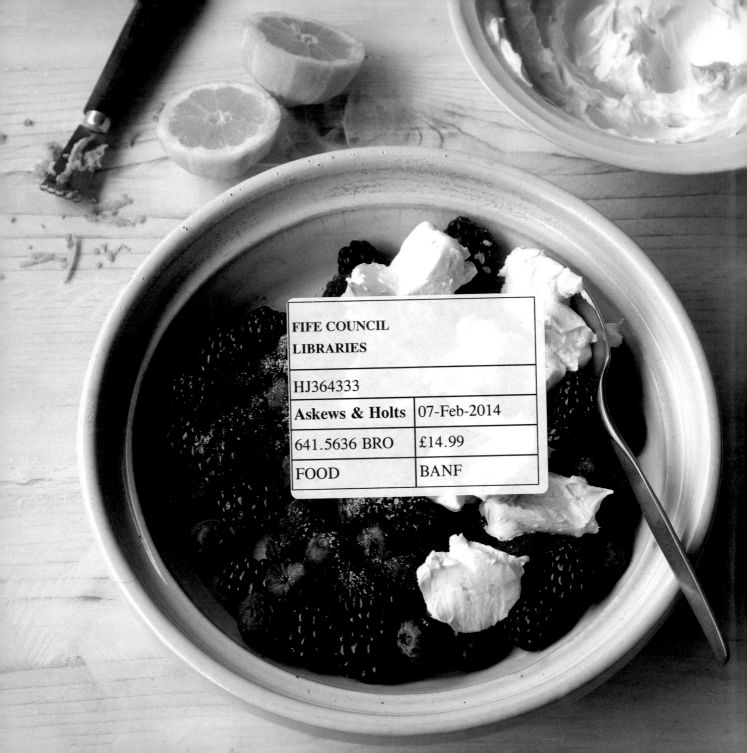

contents

introduction

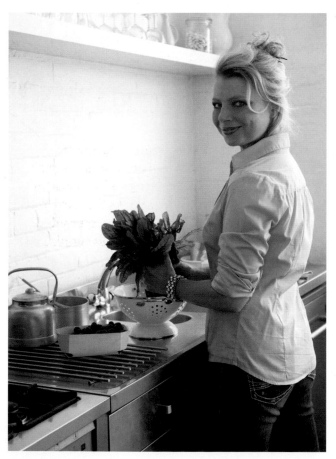

"Have you heard about this great new diet? No third helpings." Stanley Kubrick

It was Stanley Kubrick's wife Christiane who first got me started on this book, nearly ten years ago when I wrote the original version. Back then, I was cooking for her, her family and friends nearly every week, so when several of them decided to try a low-carb diet, it was time for me to get my low-carb thinking cap on. This is the result of many months' experimenting, learning, feasting, and losing weight!

This is not a diet book, it's a cookbook. That said, it's a cookbook mainly for those who have embraced the low-carb lifestyle that is set to dominate the Western world in the 21st century, especially as refined carbs and sugars become more and more demonised by health experts. The low-carb diet has undergone criticism, but there's no doubt it works for those who stick to it. Surely obesity is more dangerous? There's an awful lot of conflicting information out there, but one point nutritionists will agree on: controlling carbs reduces appetite, and if you eat less, you will lose weight.

To be true to this project, I went on a low-carb diet myself. I had been a normal, healthy weight for several years and didn't have much weight to lose, but I have had plump phases in my life and I know how fabulous it feels to get thin. What I really wanted was to "live the low-carb life" to get a clearer picture of what the diet is really like. I was surprised! Almost immediately, I noticed that my appetite shrank. I was snacking less and eating smaller meals. I really did feel that my mind was more focused and I had sustained energy levels. I could sit at my desk for hours without even thinking about what I would wander into the kitchen to nibble on next. Unlike other diets, there was not a sense of deprivation or longing. After two weeks, my clothes felt loose and I had lost about 3 lbs. This proved to me that the diet works.

I think it's the stereotype of the "fat chef" that often prompts people to ask me, "How do you stay so slim?" My reply is always the same. "Plenty of exercise!" Whatever diet you're on, that's the key. I advise anyone embarking on a low-carb diet to read the books that are out there and decide what's right for them. Pair that up with increased physical exercise, and you have nothing to lose but excess weight.

Developing these recipes was a whole new experience for me. I established a finite set of ingredients that were low-carb and vegetarian. Within that realm, I applied the same passion and relish as I always do, aiming to create the most sumptuous dishes I could muster. I hope this cookbook will contribute some ideas to your repertoire, vegetarian or not, low-carb or not, and that the recipes are as fun to cook as they are to eat. It's good food – enjoy!

Celia Brooks, 2013

how it works

There are two factors that make the low-carb diet unique: The first is insulin control. When you eat carbohydrates, the body quickly converts them into the basic sugars of which they are composed. The presence of these sugars in the bloodstream gives you a surge of energy, but also triggers the pancreas to produce insulin. Insulin's job is to enter the bloodstream and remove the sugars for storage as fat. This happens fast, and once the insulin has stored the sugars, your appetite returns. It follows that if you eat fewer carbs, your body doesn't have the sugars there to burn for fuel, so it resorts to the fat stores, and off drops the excess weight.

The second factor is how protein affects appetite. Carbs burn up quickly; protein takes longer to digest. So a high-protein meal, with plenty of tofu or eggs, for example, will leave you feeling fuller for longer. You are then less likely to snack between meals and end up eating less. If you do fancy a snack, you'll get more mileage out of a high-protein one.

Protein is the obvious stumbling block for a vegetarian on a low-carb diet. It is assumed that the diet is too limiting without meat or fish. While it would be impossible to follow a no-carb diet as a veggie (and this would be discouraged from a health point of view), there are plenty of high-protein, low-carb options available, especially eggs and tofu, and they both dominate the recipes in this book. Because of the high vegetable content of many of the recipes, I would argue that going low-carb vegetarian could be one of the healthiest diets around. After all, vegetables are the elixir of life.

PROTEIN

Protein is your best friend on a low-carb diet. Many vegetarian protein sources, except nuts and cheese, are also low in fat, which increases your chances of successful weight loss. Not only that, but all natural vegetarian protein sources are rich in other nutrients that can improve your general health. Beans and legumes are protein-rich, but they are also carb-rich. Having set myself the challenge of creating recipes with just 10 g carbs or less per serving, I found it best to leave these out of the recipes, but, along with wholegrains, they should form part of a balanced diet and can be consumed in moderation if you are not being too strict with your carb count.

EGGS

Eggs are often referred to as "the perfect protein". As with all other animal protein sources, they contain all twenty amino acids that form a complete protein, all wrapped up in a neat little shell. Eggs contain many beneficial minerals and vitamins, including vitamin E – a natural antioxidant which helps prevent disease. While the belief has long been held that the cholesterol in eggs is unhealthy, doctors and health organisations no longer advise restricting egg consumption. Studies have found no relationship between dietary cholesterol or egg consumption and heart disease risk.

I can't stress enough the importance of buying organic eggs. Not only do organic chickens have a happier life in their free-range surroundings, but their diet is totally vegetarian and free of chemicals, antibiotics and hormones. On a low-carb vegetarian diet, your egg intake will be high. Since what goes into the chicken goes into the egg, which then goes into you, organic is the only way to go. Yes, they are a little bit more expensive, but only by a fraction, well worth spending.

SOYA

The mighty soybean is Nature's gift to vegetarians. It is one of the only plant sources of complete protein (as with animal protein, it too contains all twenty amino acids). Soybean products are low in fat and carbs, high in protein and disease-preventing antioxidants, and also high in plant oestrogens which have many benefits, including reducing the risk of breast cancer. In fact, the USFDA recommends that everyone incorporate at least 25 g soya protein into their daily diet, to help reduce cholesterol levels. While most natural foods lose their good qualities and nutrients in processing, the opposite is true of soya. A cake of processed tofu has more concentrated nutrients than the raw bean, and fewer carbs weight for weight. As with eggs, organic soya is best. Be aware that non-organic soya is often genetically modified.

NUTS

Nuts and seeds are powerhouses of nutrition. They are high in protein and also boast a high vitamin E, fibre and mineral content. Brazil nuts contain high levels of selenium, which is particularly beneficial for vegetarians as it's one of the only plant sources of this essential mineral. Nuts score high in the fat department, but it's good, unsaturated fat. Walnuts are one of the few plant sources of omega-3 fats, the cholesterol-lowering fats found in oily fish.

DAIRY

Although dairy products do contain saturated fat, this is no longer considered harmful. Even saturated fats are crucial for health and do not raise heart disease risk. There are many low-fat dairy products available, but they almost always contain a higher carb count. 100 g/3½ fl oz of low-fat yogurt contains 7.4 g carbs, while the same quantity of thick and creamy Greek-style yogurt contains just 4.8 g. Reduced-fat crème fraîche generally contains zero or very low carbs, so I've used that in some of the recipes.

As a general rule of thumb, the higher the fat content of the dairy item, the lower the carbs – butter and most cheeses contain none. All dairy foods are products – they have been processed – so always check the nutritional information on the packaging, in case some carbs have sneaked in. Also, not all cheeses are strictly vegetarian, as animal rennet is used in the manufacturing. There are quite a few recipes here using Parmesan, and a proper Italian *Parmigiano Reggiano* will have been made using animal rennet. There are some very good vegetarian Parmesan substitutes out there, so please seek them out. When buying any of the cheeses used in this book, please check the label to make sure it's vegetarian if that is a concern for you.

FIBRE

One criticism by nutritionists of low-carb diets is the lack of fibre, which is essential to keep the digestive system on track. A vegetarian low-carb diet is safe from this worry, provided you eat plenty of the permitted low-carb vegetables used in this book.

SUGAR

This is the BIG no-no. All sugars, refined or not, are pure carbohydrate and will send your insulin levels soaring and throw your metabolism off kilter if you are maintaining a strict low-carb lifestyle. Low-calorie sweetener is the low-carb alternative. All recipes in this book that contain a sweet element were developed using Splenda® brand granulated sweetener, a sucralose-based product (see www.splenda.com for more information). Canderel Yellow® Granular is another sucralose product available in the UK. These products are derived from sugar but have virtually no calories or carbs and do not affect insulin levels. Unlike some sweeteners, they are suitable for cooking and will stay sweet when subjected to heat. They do have a bit of an aftertaste, but seem to taste more authentic when an acidic element such as lemon is introduced, as is true of some other sugar-free sweeteners. Have you noticed how a squeeze of lemon improves the flavour of diet cola?

If you prefer not to use a sucralose product, you could try an alternative such as xylitol, or a stevia-based sweetener such as Truvia® or Canderel Green®. Please bear in mind that use of these sweeteners might require changing the quantities used in the recipes, so check the products' packaging and recommendations on their websites.

In the Sweet Things chapter, I have used highest-quality diabetic chocolate for some recipes. This chocolate is sweetened with sugar alcohols such as maltitol or sorbitol. Look for stockists online, in health-food shops and pharmacies.

FAT

Fats, like carbs, are often misunderstood – it is a blanket generalisation to assume they are all bad. There are good fats and bad fats. Plant sources are good fats. Good fats, from plant sources – monounsaturated, polyunsaturated and omegas – are an essential part of our diet and actually lower cholesterol. Animal fats, including eggs and dairy, were once considered bad fats, but in fact they are good for health. They do not raise cholesterol and clog the arteries as once thought. The worst offenders are trans fats – highly processed solid fats used in certain margarines and processed foods – which have been proven dangerous. Always check labels on processed foods and avoid anything that contains the word "hydrogenated" in the ingredients.

Fat contains twice the calories of carbs, so it seems logical that if you cut out fat, you'll lose calories and hence weight, but this is a misconception which led to an obsession with avoiding fat. As with carbs, the trick is actually to avoid the bad and enjoy the good, and as with all things, in moderation.

CARBS

Not all carbs are your enemy. There are evil carbs and angelic ones. Generally, the bad guys are the white, refined carbs: white bread, white pasta, potatoes, white rice and white sugar. These are the foods that will give you a surge of energy followed by a crash and a new wave of hunger pangs, potentially leading to progressive munching, bingeing and weight gain. To make matters worse, they have few nutritional benefits otherwise. The good guys are the unrefined carbs: whole grains, including brown rice, wholemeal pasta, fruits and vegetables. These are essential for a healthy diet. Grain products are not included in this book, as I strove to keep each recipe under 10 g of carbs.

If you are looking for substitutes for pasta, noodles and rice, there are some fantastic carb-free and low-carb substitutes available online and in speciality shops. Traditional Asian shirataki noodles are virtually carb-free and calorie-free and are a natural product made from a root called konjac. There are several types of noodles and "rice" made from konjac. Follow packet directions carefully when cooking.

GLUTEN

Since I have avoided all wheat and most grain products in creating the recipes for this book, by default, every recipe is gluten-free. Obviously, if you are following a strict gluten-free diet, you should check the label on any manufactured ingredients to be sure they are suitable for you. There are a number of recipes that use soy sauce, so make sure you choose a gluten-free version, such as a Japanese tamari (shoyu is made using wheat and soy).

THE LAST WORD... WATER

Drinking water is one of the most important parts of weight loss and daily function generally. It flushes out toxins, gives a feeling of fullness, speeds up weight loss and keeps every cell in your body functioning properly. Keep a bottle with you at all times and drink at least 2 litres/3½ pints a day.

GUIDELINES FOR A HEALTHY LOW-CARB DIET

- Eat the right carbs: plenty of permitted vegetables and wholefoods. Avoid refined carbs and sugars.

- Increase your lean protein intake. At each meal, make the protein portion the larger one, the carb portion the smaller one, and always include fresh vegetables.

- As well as eating your greens, take a multivitamin and mineral supplement.

- Don't worry about saturated fat. It's trans fats and sugars that you need to avoid.

- Relax and enjoy cooking. Bon appétit!

the low-carb kitchen

If you are committing to a low-carb diet, then it's a good idea to have a "carb cull" and remove all temptation from your kitchen. Gather all high-carb foods and give to friends or donate them to charity. If other members of your household are still eating carbs, then designate a "carb cupboard" for them and stash their ingredients away; out of sight, out of mind.

Outlined in the next few pages is a selection of foods that are acceptable on the diet. Keeping a well-stocked kitchen will make the diet easy to follow and the cooking more enjoyable. In the case of fresh produce, do try to buy what's in season close to the time you want to cook it, and buy organic where possible.

* = READ THE LABEL
Products containing sugar, corn syrup, modified starch, and anything hydrogenated should be avoided.

DAIRY

- Cheese, cream cheese
- Cottage cheese
- Ricotta, mascarpone
- Butter
- Crème fraîche/sour cream, regular or reduced fat
- Whipping cream
- Semi-skimmed milk
- Thick/Greek/low-fat yogurt

EGGS

- Buy organic
- Store in the fridge

TOFU

- Firm – store in the fridge. Unused portions can be stored covered in fresh water in the fridge for up to 3 days, changing the water daily. Can be frozen
- Silken – usually sold in a long-life carton; suitable for smoothies and desserts. Unused portions should be stored in the fridge and used within 24 hours
- Smoked – store in the fridge. Can be frozen
- Flavoured*/marinated* – store in the fridge. Can be frozen

SOYA/VEGETARIAN PRODUCTS, DRIED, CHILLED OR FROZEN

- Soy flour (defatted) – store in fridge
- Textured vegetable protein (TVP)*
- Vegetarian mince*
- Quorn™ and Quorn™ products*
- Vegetarian hot dogs*, sausages*
- Soya bacon bits* and strips*
- Vegetarian deli meat such as sliced "ham" and "chicken"*

NUTS/SEEDS

- All types. Store in airtight container in a cool place for a short period, or in the freezer for longer periods. Cashew nuts are the only relatively high-carb nuts, but fine in moderation

SPICES

- All types. Store away from sunlight. Buy whole spices and grind fresh if possible. Check the label of spice mixtures which might contain sugar

CONDIMENTS/ FLAVOURINGS

- Sugar-free sweetener (recipes in this book have been developed using granulated Splenda® – see pp.9–10)
- Sea salt
- Almond extract*
- Pure vanilla extract*
- Tabasco® sauce
- Other chilli sauces*
- Soy sauce (such as a gluten-free tamari), light and dark
- Mustard*, dry and prepared
- Mayonnaise*
- Peanut butter*
- Cooking wines: sherry, Madeira, Marsala

TINS/CANS/JARS

- Italian chopped tomatoes
- Artichoke hearts/bottoms
- Pickled vegetables*
- Pickled chillies such as jalapeños*
- Green and black olives
- Capers
- Roasted peppers*
- Water chestnuts
- Palm hearts
- Coconut milk/cream

- Pesto*
- Tapenade*

FRESH PRODUCE

- All green vegetables and salad
- Cauliflower
- Spring onions, shallots, onions, garlic, leeks
- Aubergines
- Pumpkin
- Asparagus
- Courgettes
- Celeriac, swede, turnips
- Capsicum peppers
- Mung bean sprouts and other sprouted seeds such as alfalfa
- Avocados
- Cucumber
- Celery
- Fennel
- Green beans, mange tout, sugar snaps
- Mushrooms of all types, fresh and dried
- Radishes
- Tomatoes
- Red and green chillies
- Ginger
- Lemons, limes
- Fresh berries, melon

DRINKS

- Natural mineral water – drink 2 litres/3½ pints a day
- Herbal tea (sweetened with sugar-free sweetener only)
- Tea/coffee
- White wine
- Vodka and some other spirits*
- Sugar-free mixers/carbonated drinks*

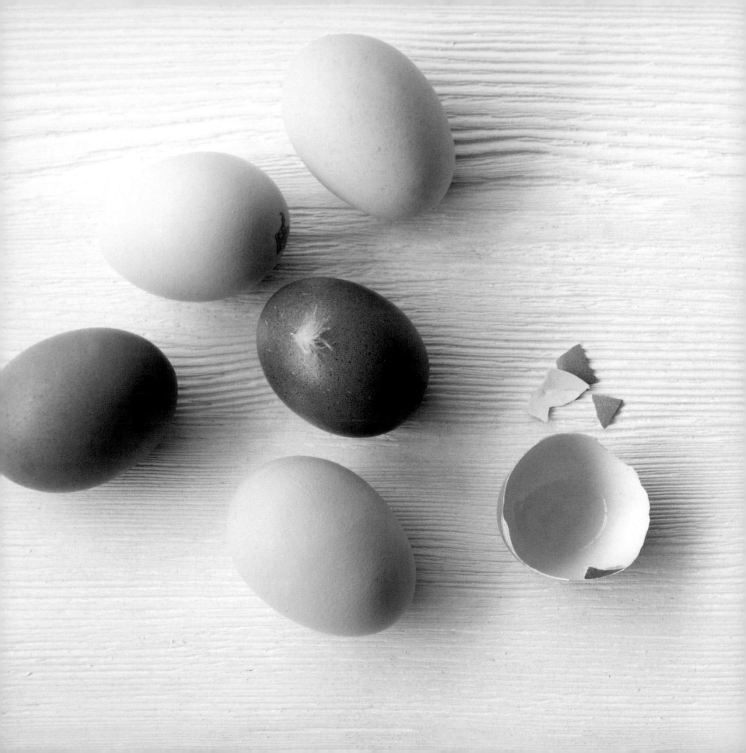

01:

BREAK FAST

A high-protein fuel injection at breakfast will rocket-propel you into a sustained orbit until lunchtime. Breakfast is the key to keeping hunger at bay throughout the day. Don't miss it...

Blueberry Almond
Griddle Cakes

These US Southern-style pancakes are sweet, nutty and laced with bursting blueberries. Don't be confused by putting the berries in the pan before the batter – it is the best way to distribute and cook them evenly, rather than mixing them into the batter.

6 tbsp soy flour

4 tbsp ground almonds

2 tbsp sweetener

½ tsp baking powder

Pinch of salt

2 eggs

50 ml/2 fl oz double cream

2 tsp butter

75 g/3 oz blueberries

2 tbsp Greek yogurt,
    to serve (optional)

Makes 12/Serves 4

Preheat the oven to 120°C/250°F/Gas Mark ½ for keeping the griddle cakes warm. Place the soy flour, almonds, sweetener, baking powder, salt, eggs and double cream in a blender and process until smooth.

Heat a large non-stick pan or griddle over a low to medium flame and add 1 tsp of the butter. Tilt the pan to coat the surface with the melted butter. Allowing 4–5 blueberries for each griddle cake, place a cluster of berries in three places in the pan and carefully pour the batter over them to make three griddle cakes about 6 cm/2½ inches in diameter. Cook until risen, golden on the undersides and dry around the edges, then flip over and cook the other sides until golden. Keep warm in the oven while you cook the remaining batches, adding the remaining butter between batches. Serve warm with the yogurt, if you like.

Per serving
Carbs: 5 g protein: 11 g calories: 267 fibre: 3 g fat: 23 g (saturated fat: 8 g)

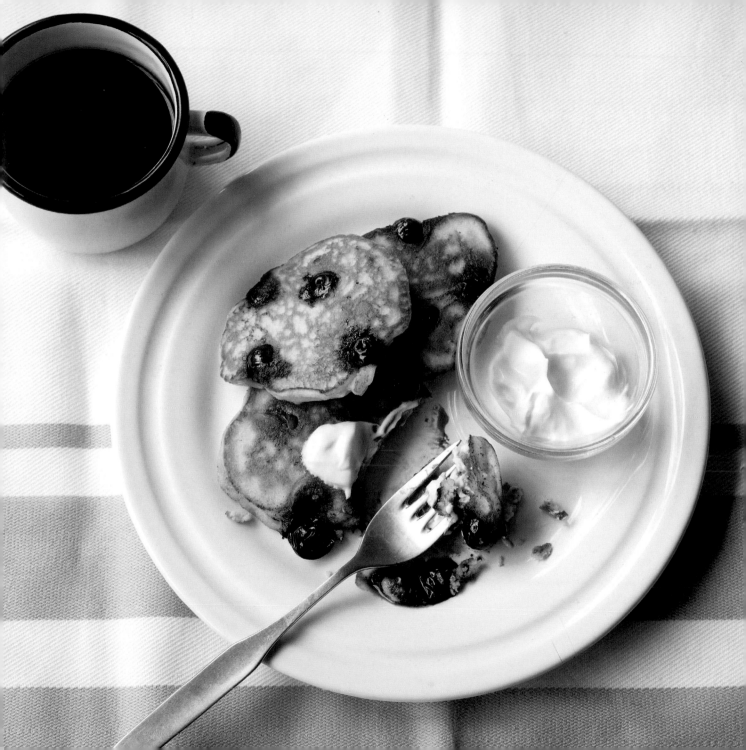

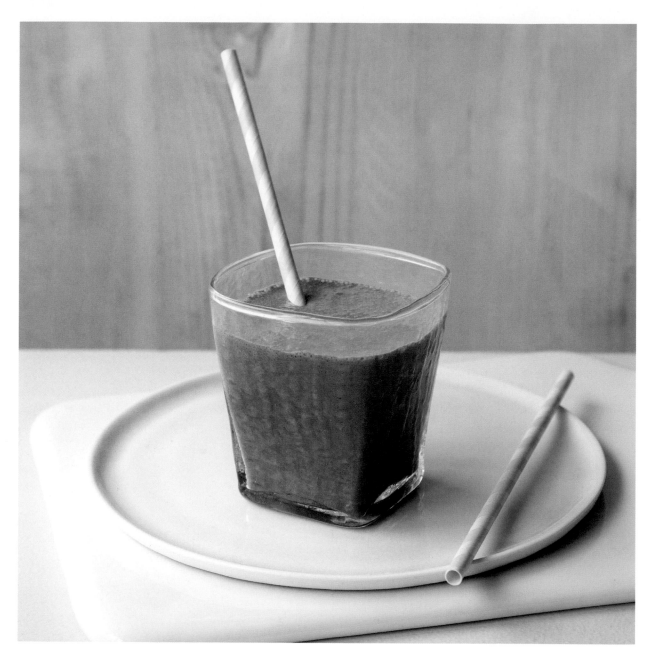

Chocolate Breakfast Shake

Chocolate for breakfast? Why not? Pure cocoa powder contains beneficial antioxidants, you get a little pro-biotic culture from the yogurt, and tofu is loaded with protein, so this delicious sugar-free shake is healthier than you might think.

150 g/5 oz silken tofu

2 tbsp Greek yogurt

200 ml/7 fl oz water

2 tbsp pure cocoa powder

½ tsp pure vanilla extract

large pinch ground cinnamon, or to taste

3 tbsp sweetener, or to taste

Serves 2

Place all ingredients in a blender and process until smooth. Taste for sweetness and add more sweetener to suit. For a thicker texture, use less water in the mixture.

Per serving

Carbs: 2 g protein: 7 g calories: 78 fibre: 0.5 g fat: 5 g (saturated fat: 1.5 g)

Melon Berry Power Smoothie

Blast off with this fruity, high-protein concoction – guaranteed to give your day a kick start.

150 g/5 oz silken tofu

50 g/2 oz cantaloupe melon chunks

50 g/2 oz raspberries

3 tbsp ground almonds

½ tsp almond extract

1 tsp mixed spice, or to taste

2 tbsp sweetener, or to taste

5 tbsp water

Serves 2

Place all ingredients in a blender and process until smooth. Taste for sweetness and add more sweetener to suit.

Per serving

Carbs: 7.5 g protein: 11 g calories: 217 fibre: 3 g fat: 16 g (saturated fat: 1.5 g)

Turkish Breakfast

A satisfying, summery collection of tasty morsels, this traditional breakfast brings the essence of the Mediterranean to your table first thing in the morning. Boiling the egg in this fashion gives it a "buttery" yolk – not too runny, nor too powdery, but just right. This recipe serves per person, but you can multiply it any number of times. Strong black tea is the customary accompaniment.

1 organic egg

25 g/1 oz slice feta cheese, crumbled
    into chunks

1 medium tomato, quartered

75 g/3 oz cucumber, cut into chunks

50 g/2 oz good-quality black olives,
    such as Kalamata

1 tbsp olive oil

½ tsp dried oregano,
    or 1 tsp fresh oregano

Salt and freshly ground black pepper

Serves 1

Place the egg in a pan and cover with cold water. Bring to the boil, then simmer for 7 minutes. Drain and rinse under cold water until cool. Crack and remove the shell and cut the egg in half – it should be set but the yolk should still be buttery.

Toss the remaining ingredients, place on a plate, and top with the egg. Drizzle the olive oil over the mixture, sprinkle with oregano and season with salt and pepper.

Per serving

Carbs: 3 g protein: 13 g calories: 318 fibre: 2.5 g fat: 28 g (saturated fat: 8 g)

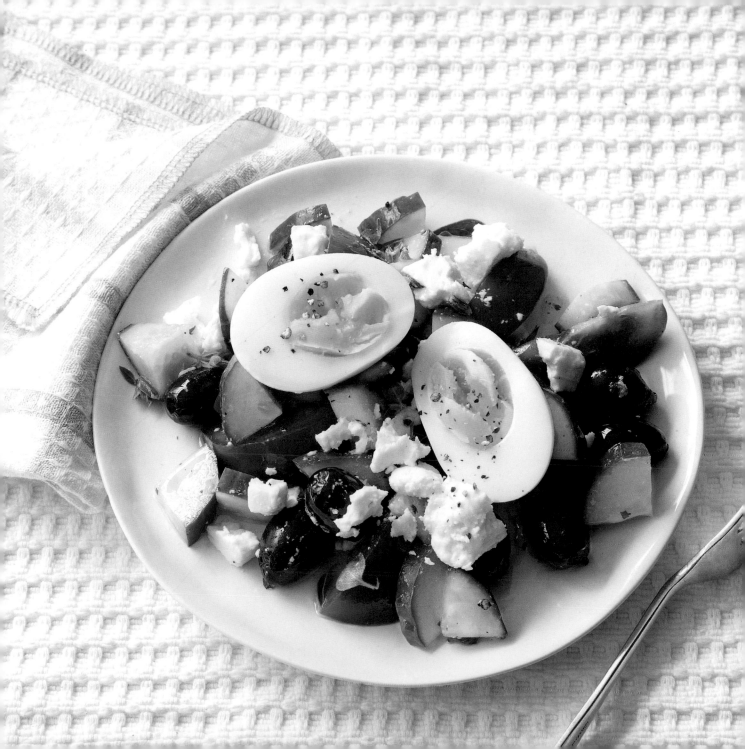

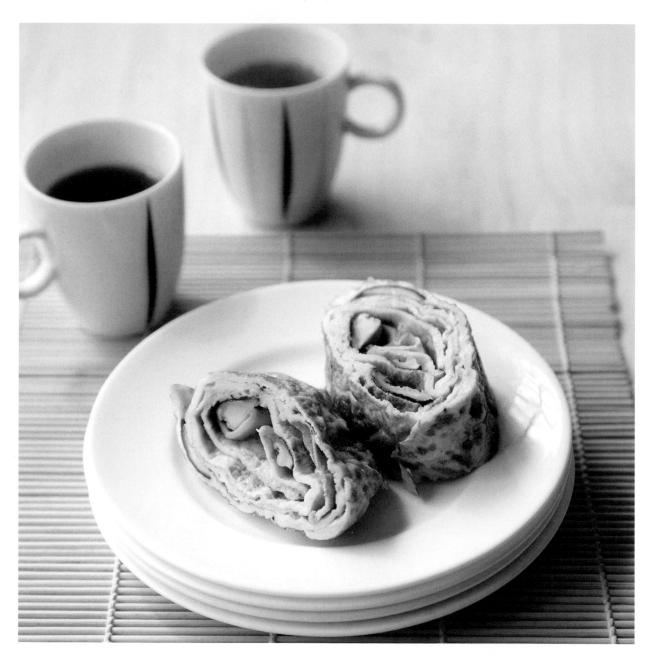

Japanese Omelette

Making this light, multi-layered, rolled omelette might take a little practice, but the result is mightily impressive. As you are making it, don't worry if some of the layers break up slightly, as they will repair themselves in the final step. The added mushrooms give the omelette a rich nutty flavour, but they are not essential. Can be made up to 1 hour in advance.

6 shiitake mushrooms
1 tbsp vegetable oil
8 organic eggs
120 ml/4 fl oz Vegetable Stock
    (see p.162)
1 tbsp light soy sauce

Serves 4

Discard the stems of the shiitake mushrooms and slice very thinly. Heat a large non-stick pan over a medium heat and add 2 tsp of the oil. Cook the mushrooms until they are tinged with gold, then drain on kitchen paper.

Beat the eggs with remaining ingredients in a jug. Reheat the pan with the remaining oil over a low to medium heat and pour in just enough of the egg mixture to cover the base, swirling to coat. Sprinkle with a few mushrooms. Cook until barely set but not dry, then loosen the edges with a spatula and fold over three or four times to one side of the pan. (It may help to use a wide fish slice, two spatulas or chopsticks.)

Pour in a little more egg mixture, swirl to coat the pan and allow the mixture to attach itself to the cooked omelette. Sprinkle on a few mushrooms and cook until barely set. Loosen as before and roll up in the opposite direction, starting with the previously cooked omelette.

Pour in more egg and mushrooms, and repeat the process, back and forth, until the egg mixture is used up and you have a long "sausage" of omelette.

Spread out a large piece of foil. Slide the omelette into the middle and roll up in the foil, gently forming it into a firm brick shape. Keep warm until ready to serve, then unwrap on a board and cut into eight slices or four pieces.

Per serving
Carbs: 0.3g protein: 16 g calories: 216 fibre: 0.5 g fat: 17 g (saturated fat: 4 g)

Kerala-Style Eggs

My cooking is heavily influenced by India, partly because it's a vegetarian's paradise, but also because I have spent some time in Kerala, the southern-most state. This is my version of one of my favourite Keralan breakfast dishes. First frying the black or brown mustard seeds gives the eggs an authentic and wonderful nuttiness, but if you can't find them, don't worry – just leave out that step, and start by frying the onions, chillies, etc.

4 organic eggs

1 tbsp sunflower oil

½ tsp black or brown mustard seeds

2 spring onions, chopped

1 fresh red chilli, sliced or chopped
    (deseeded if large)

½ tsp finely grated fresh root ginger

½ tsp ground turmeric

1 tomato, about 100 g/3½ oz, chopped

Handful of fresh coriander, chopped

Salt and freshly ground black pepper

2 tsp Greek yogurt, to serve (optional)

Serves 2

Beat the eggs in a bowl with a large pinch of salt until frothy. Set aside.

Heat a non-stick frying pan over a medium to high heat and pour in the oil. Add the mustard seeds and when they start to pop, lower the heat. Add the spring onions and chilli and cook for about 1 minute, until fragrant. Add the ginger and turmeric and stir, then add tomatoes and cook for about 1 minute more.

When the tomatoes are heated through, pour in the eggs. When the eggs have set on the base of the pan, start stirring gently with a folding motion. Cook until nearly set, then stir in the coriander and remove from the heat. Serve on warm plates with a spoonful of yogurt and plenty of freshly ground black pepper.

Per serving
Carbs: 2.5 g protein: 16 g calories: 240 fibre: 0.7 g fat: 19 g (saturated fat: 5 g)

Three-Minute Egg and Mushroom Bowl

The microwave is brilliant for cooking vegetables with a high water content such as mushrooms. This recipe is so speedy it might well be the fastest low-carb breakfast in the West! The recipe is for one, but of course it can be multiplied – although it's best to cook each portion individually.

1 large flat field (portobello)
    mushroom, stem removed
1 tsp truffle oil or olive oil
1 egg
Sea salt and freshly ground
    black pepper
25 g/1 oz Cheddar or other mature,
    tangy cheese, cut into 2 slices
1 tsp bacon-flavour soya bits
    (optional)

Serves 1

Choose a microwave-safe bowl that is just wide enough to accommodate the mushroom cap but not much bigger. Place the mushroom cap, gill side up, in the bowl. Drizzle the truffle oil or olive oil over the gills and season with salt and pepper. (You could also add a little chopped garlic or fresh herbs at this stage.)

Break the egg into the mushroom. Season lightly and prick the yolk with a fork to prevent it from exploding. Cross the cheese slices on top. Sprinkle over the bacon-flavour soya bits, if using.

Microwave on high for 1 minute, then check. The cooking time is variable (1½–2 minutes), depending on the moisture content and size of the mushroom, the size of the egg, the power of the microwave, etc. It's best to judge by the cheese, which should be bubbly and slightly crisp. The egg white should be completely set.

Per serving
Carbs: 0.2 g protein: 15 g calories: 223 fibre: 0.4 g fat: 18 g (saturated fat: 8 g)

Eggs Florentine
with Grilled Mushrooms

Juicy, truffle-scented field (portobello) mushrooms replace English muffins in this timeless classic – a fabulous brunch dish. A little multitasking is required, but it's worth it. Warm plates are absolutely essential for serving – pop them in the base of the oven while the mushrooms are cooking. If you don't have a grill, simply roast the mushrooms at 200°C/400°F/Gas Mark 6 instead.

4 large, flat field
    (portobello) mushrooms
2 tbsp olive oil
2 tsp truffle oil (optional)
4 organic eggs
400 g/14 oz young spinach leaves
1 quantity Blender Hollandaise
    (see p.164)
Salt and freshly ground black pepper

Serves 4

First, cook the mushrooms. Preheat the grill to its highest setting. Snap the stems out of the mushrooms and discard. Brush the caps with olive oil and place, gill side up, on a baking sheet. Season with salt and pepper, and drizzle the remaining olive oil and truffle oil, if using, over the gills. Place under the grill for about 8 minutes, until juicy. Keep warm.

Meanwhile, poach the eggs. Bring a 2 cm/¾ inch depth of water to the boil in a large, non-stick frying pan. Lower the heat to a gentle simmer. One at a time, carefully break each egg into a cup, then slide it into the water. Simmer for 2 minutes. Turn off the heat and leave the eggs to stand in the water for 10 minutes for slightly runny yolks. If you prefer a well-done yolk, return the pan to the heat for 1–2 minutes, until cooked to your liking. Place a couple of layers of kitchen paper on a plate. Remove the eggs from the pan with a slotted spatula and dry briefly on the paper. Keep warm.

Place the spinach in a large, heatproof bowl and pour boiling water over it. Stir until wilted, then drain thoroughly in a sieve or colander, pressing out the excess moisture with a potato masher. Keep the spinach warm while you make the hollandaise sauce, which ideally should be made just before serving, but can also be made ahead and reheated.

Place a grilled mushroom cap on each of four warm plates. Top with spinach, then a poached egg. Finish with warm hollandaise sauce and a good grinding of black pepper.

Per serving
Carbs: 2.5 g protein: 14 g calories: 499 fibre: 3 g fat: 48 g (saturated fat: 23 g)

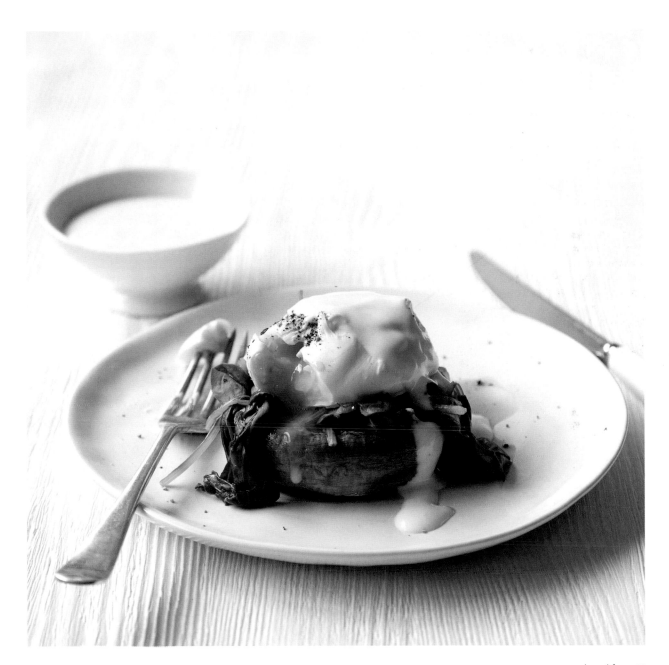

Cottage Cheese Scramble

This recipe produces the tastiest and easiest scrambled eggs, all done in just three minutes. The wonderful cottage cheese imparts a richness and texture that makes toast just seem irrelevant. You can supplement this breakfast with a veggie sausage or two (low-carb ones, of course – always read the label), cooked in the microwave for speed and ease.

4 eggs

4 tbsp cottage cheese, drained

Sea salt and freshly ground
    black pepper

1 tsp butter

Serves 2

Whisk together the eggs, cottage cheese and seasoning in a bowl. Heat a non-stick frying pan over a low heat and add the butter. Pour in the eggs. Cook until the underside is just set, then stir gently until the whole mixture is just set. Serve immediately.

(This can also be cooked in a microwave: Place the egg mixture in a microwave-safe bowl and add the butter. Cook on high power for 1 minute, then stir. Cook for a further 1–2 minutes, stopping and stirring with a clean fork every minute until cooked to your liking.)

Per serving
Carbs: 1 g protein: 19 g calories: 228 fibre: 0 g fat: 17 g (saturated fat: 6 g)

Cottage Cheese Pancakes
with Berry Purée

A short-stack of these classic American-style pancakes makes a filling breakfast. They can also be frozen (after cooking and cooling), then reheated in a toaster straight from the freezer.

2 tbsp soy flour
1 tsp sweetener
100 g/3½ oz cottage cheese
2 eggs, beaten
½ tsp baking powder
Generous pinch of sea salt
1 tsp sunflower oil
Raspberry Purée (see p.165),
    to serve

Serves 2

Preheat the oven to about 120°C/250°F/Gas Mark ½ to keep the pancakes warm once cooked.

Beat together the flour, sweetener, cottage cheese, eggs, baking powder and salt until well mixed, making sure there are no lumps of flour.

Heat a large non-stick frying pan over a medium heat and add the oil. Cook tablespoonfuls of the mixture in batches. When golden underneath, flip the pancakes over carefully – they remain slightly runnier on top than standard pancakes. Cook the second side, then remove to a plate and keep warm while you cook another batch.

Serve warm with Raspberry Purée spooned on top of each pancake.

Per serving
Carbs: 5 g protein: 17 g calories: 194 fibre: 2 g fat: 12 g (saturated fat: 3.5 g)

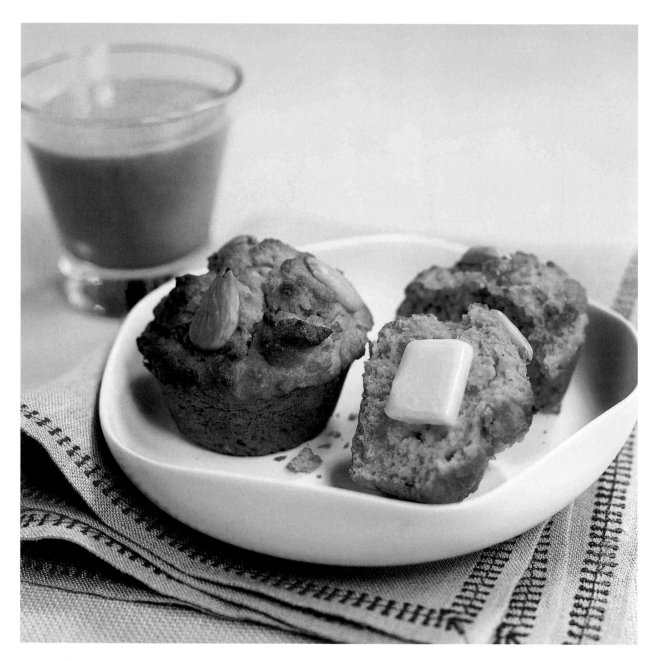

Almond Muffins

These protein-packed muffins are easy to grab and eat on busy mornings. This recipe makes a large batch, but they keep well for up to four days in an airtight container or can be frozen. Alternatively, you can divide the recipe in half or into thirds, if you want to make less.

For the dry mixture
225 g/8 oz soy flour
150 g/5 oz ground almonds
3 tsp baking powder
15 tbsp sweetener
1 tsp salt

For the wet mixture
6 eggs, beaten
135 ml/4½ fl oz reduced-fat
    crème fraîche or sour cream
1 tbsp vanilla extract
1½ tsp almond extract
135 ml/4½ fl oz sunflower oil

To decorate and serve
36 blanched almonds
butter

Makes 12

Preheat oven to 180°C/350°F/Gas Mark 4. Grease a 12-cup muffin tin or line with paper cases and set aside.

Combine all the dry ingredients in a bowl, smoothing out any lumps in the flour.

Beat together all the wet ingredients in another bowl. Thoroughly combine the two mixtures, but do not over-mix.

Pour the batter into the prepared muffin tin. Place 3 blanched almonds on top of each. Bake for 20–30 minutes, until risen, golden and firm. Rest for 5 minutes in the tin, then turn out onto a wire rack. Serve warm, with butter for spreading.

Per serving
Carbs: 6 g protein: 14 g calories: 298 fibre: 3 g fat: 24 g (saturated fat: 4 g)

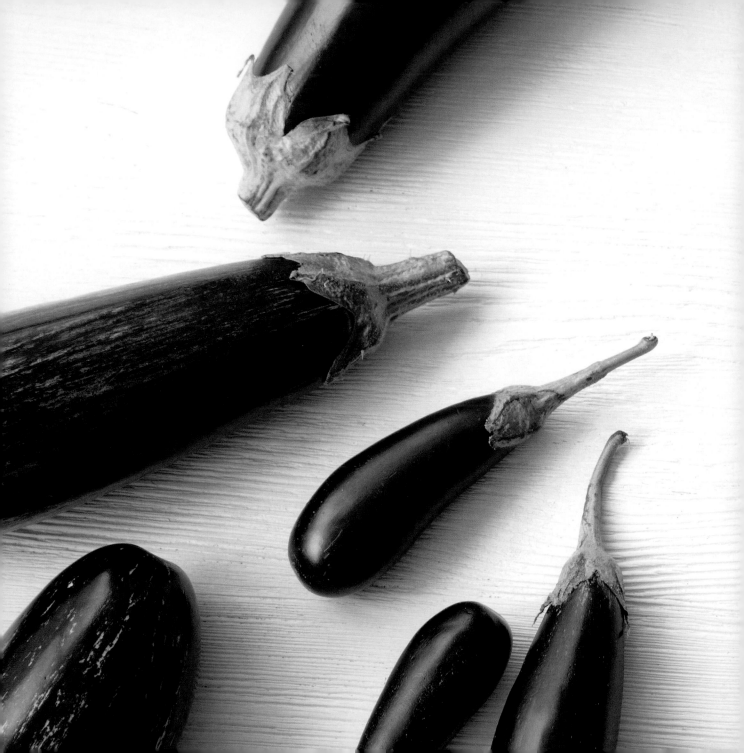

02:
SMALL
COURSES

These little dishes can be mixed and matched with other recipes from this book, for a table full of treats, the prelude to a main course, instalments in a multi-course feast, or served as a single light meal.

Fragrant Coconut Broth

Here's the closest thing you can possibly get to fresh coconut milk – an easy method of reconstituting dried coconut, then pressing out the milk. You'll be amazed how light and refreshing it tastes. If you are short of time, use a standard (400 ml/14 oz) tin of coconut milk plus 600 ml/1 pint water or vegetable stock instead.

250 g/9 oz desiccated coconut
    (unsweetened)
1.25 litres/2 pints boiling water
4 cm/1½ inch piece of fresh root
    ginger, peeled
2 lemongrass stalks, trimmed
2 tbsp light soy sauce, or to taste
1 tbsp sweetener
50 g/2 oz button mushrooms, sliced
50 g/2 oz broccoli florets, chopped
1 tbsp lemon juice
Handful of fresh coriander leaves
    (optional)

Serves 4

Place the coconut in a bowl, pour over the boiling water and leave to cool. When cold, purée with a hand-held or upright blender, then push through a sieve, squeezing out as much coconut milk as possible; there should be just under 1 litre/1¾ pints.

Slice the ginger and lemongrass – doing this now will maximise the flavour (as opposed to slicing ahead of time). Place in a pan with the coconut milk, soy sauce and sweetener.

Bring to the boil, lower the heat and simmer, stirring occasionally, for 10 minutes. Add the mushrooms and broccoli, return to the boil and cook for 3 minutes. Ladle the broth into small bowls. Season with a little lemon juice in each bowl, top with coriander leaves (if using) and serve.

Per serving
Carbs: 5 g protein: 5 g calories: 388 fibre: 9 g fat: 39 g (saturated fat: 33 g)

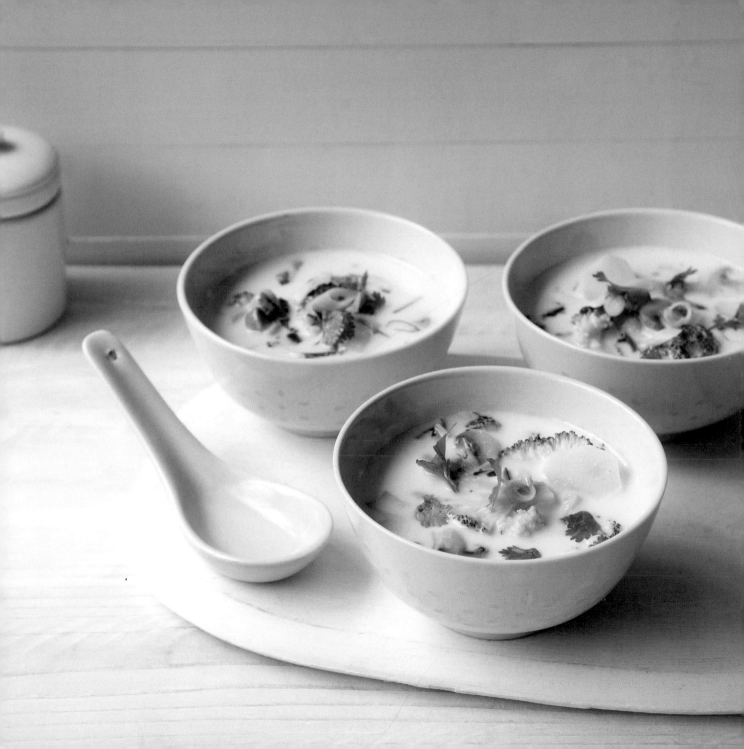

Asian Wild Mushroom Broth

Dried mushrooms such as shiitake have a concentrated flavour that is released into this light and cleansing broth, giving it a rich, nutty undertone.

1 litre/1¾ pints Vegetable Stock
    (see p.162)
10 dried shiitake mushrooms
    or other dried mushrooms,
    about 10 g/¼ oz, rinsed
1 tbsp sunflower oil
1 garlic clove, chopped
2 cm/¾ inch piece of fresh
    root ginger, chopped
100 g/3½ oz tofu, finely diced
150 g/5 oz fresh mixed wild or
    cultivated exotic mushrooms
    (such as enoki, shimeji, oyster,
    shiitake), cut into bite-size pieces
1 tbsp dark soy sauce
1 punnet, about 20 g/¾ oz, salad
    cress, such as mustard or shiso,
    or other sprouting seeds,
    trimmed and cleaned

Serves 4

Place the stock and dried mushrooms in a saucepan and bring to the boil. Simmer for at least 15 minutes. (If the shiitake mushrooms seem a little large to eat, use a pair of scissors to snip them to size in the broth, once softened. Alternatively, lift them out with a slotted spoon, leave to cool a bit, then chop and return them to the broth.)

Meanwhile, heat a small frying pan over a moderate flame and add the sunflower oil. Add garlic, ginger and tofu, and stir-fry for about 2 minutes, until fragrant but not brown. Add the fresh mushrooms and stir-fry until soft and juicy. Add the soy sauce and remove from the heat.

Empty the contents of the frying pan into the simmering stock. Bring back to a simmer for 5 minutes, then taste for seasoning. Ladle the soup into bowls, scatter cress or sprouting seeds over the top, and serve.

Per serving
Carbs: 8 g protein: 13 g calories: 141 fibre: 0.5 g fat: 7 g (saturated fat: 0.4 g)

Porcini Mushroom Soup with Thyme

Dried porcini mushrooms are a magic stock item with the power to transform the ordinary into something elegant. Cooking this velvety soup fills the house with delectable earthy aromas.

25 g/1 oz dried porcini mushrooms

600 ml/1 pint boiling Vegetable Stock (see p.162) or water

2 tbsp olive oil

3 garlic cloves, crushed

500 g/1¼ lb flat or other fresh mushrooms, coarsely chopped

1½ tsp salt

Bunch of fresh thyme, rinsed and tied together, or 1 tsp dried thyme

150 ml/¼ pint Madeira, sherry or Marsala

4 tbsp reduced-fat crème fraîche or sour cream

4 tbsp chopped parsley

Freshly ground black pepper

Serves 4

Rinse the porcini to remove any soil or grit, then place in a bowl and pour the boiling stock or water over them. Leave for 20 minutes, then strain over a bowl, reserving the liquid. Coarsely chop the porcini.

Heat the olive oil in a pan over a low to medium heat and add the garlic. Cook for just a few seconds, until it becomes fragrant, without letting it burn or colour too much. Add the chopped mushrooms and porcini and season with the salt and plenty of pepper. Stir, then cover and cook, stirring occasionally, for about 10 minutes, until the mushrooms have collapsed and are stewing in their juices.

Add the thyme and wine, then pour in the reserved mushroom soaking liquid through a fine strainer, to leave behind any extra grit which may have settled. Bring to the boil, then lower the heat to a simmer. Cook, uncovered, for 10 minutes. Cool briefly, then remove and discard the thyme bundle, if using, and purée the soup with a hand-held blender or in a food processor. Check the seasoning. The texture of the soup may vary depending on how juicy your mushrooms are; if it seems too thick, dilute with a little boiling water. Ladle into bowls and finish each with a tablespoon of crème fraîche or sour cream and chopped parsley.

Per serving

Carbs: 7 g protein: 4 g calories: 163 fibre: 1.5 g fat: 8 g (saturated fat: 2.5 g)

Egg Flower Soup

"Flower" in the title of this recipe refers to the appearance of the eggs, which resemble chrysanthemum petals as they cook in this delicious and healthy soup. The vegetables can be adapted according to what you have available – you can substitute spinach, watercress, asparagus, or courgettes, or add a little extra ginger or chilli if you like.

1 tbsp sunflower oil

100 g/3½ oz spring onions, chopped

2 tsp sesame seeds

100 g/3½ oz broccoli, chopped

100 g/3½ oz green cabbage, finely shredded

1 litre/1¾ pints Vegetable Stock (see p.162)

1 tbsp rice vinegar

1 tsp Chinese five-spice powder

3 organic eggs

2 tbsp light soy sauce

1 tbsp dry sherry

Sea salt and freshly ground black pepper

Serves 4

Heat a pan over a low to medium heat and add the oil. Add the spring onions and sesame seeds and cook for about 2 minutes, until the sesame seeds start to turn golden. Add the broccoli and cabbage (or green vegetables of your choice) and stir-fry for about 1 minute, until bright green. Pour in the stock, season with pepper and add the vinegar and five-spice. Bring to the boil.

Meanwhile, beat together the eggs, soy sauce and sherry in a jug. While stirring the boiling soup rapidly and constantly, gradually pour in the egg mixture in a steady stream. The eggs should set immediately and the soup is ready to serve.

Per serving
Carbs: 5 g protein: 9 g calories: 150 fibre: 2 g fat: 10 g (saturated fat: 2 g)

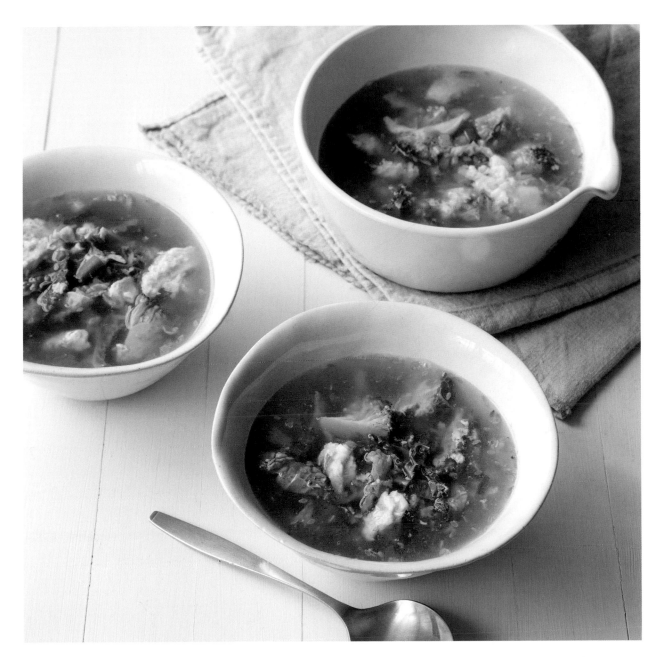

Smoky Aubergine Timbales

"Timbale" describes anything prepared in a small, round mould, either layered, as here, or solid, as in Red Pepper and Goat's Cheese Timbales (see p.45). Choose plump aubergines with about the same circumference as the ramekins, but remember that they shrink a lot when cooked. The smoky pesto has a dazzling flavour, and can be used as a sauce in other dishes (see Spaghetti Squash with Smoked Chilli Pesto, p.80).

2 large aubergines,
    about 500 g/1¼ lb total
2 garlic cloves, sliced
Olive oil
125 g/4 oz ricotta cheese
Salt and freshly ground black pepper
50 g/2 oz rocket or basil leaves,
    to garnish

For the smoky pesto
1 tsp mild smoked paprika/pimentón
Bunch of fresh basil
50 g/2 oz pine nuts
1 garlic clove
25 g/1 oz grated fresh Parmesan cheese
3 tbsp olive oil
Pinch of salt

Serves 4

Preheat the oven to 190°C/375°F/Gas Mark 5.

Slice the aubergines into 1 cm/½ inch thick rounds. Mix the garlic with some olive oil in a cup and brush both sides of the rounds. Place on a baking sheet and sprinkle the sliced garlic on top of them. Season with salt and pepper and bake for 20–30 minutes, until soft and barely golden. Leave to cool.

Make the pesto by processing all the ingredients in the food processor, adding the olive oil at the end. Taste for seasoning.

Brush 4 ramekins lightly with olive oil and place an aubergine round in each. Top with about a tablespoon of ricotta, a generous spoonful of pesto, then another aubergine round. Continue with another layer of ricotta, pesto, then aubergine. (Some pieces will be smaller than others, so use as many pieces of aubergine as necessary to fill the layer.)

Place the ramekins on a baking sheet and bake for 15–20 minutes, until sizzling. Cool briefly before inverting. To do this, place a plate upside down on top of each timbale and flip over. Remove the ramekin. Arrange rocket or basil leaves around the timbales and serve.

Per serving
Carbs: 5 g protein: 16 g calories: 541 fibre: 3 g fat: 51 g (saturated fat: 11 g)

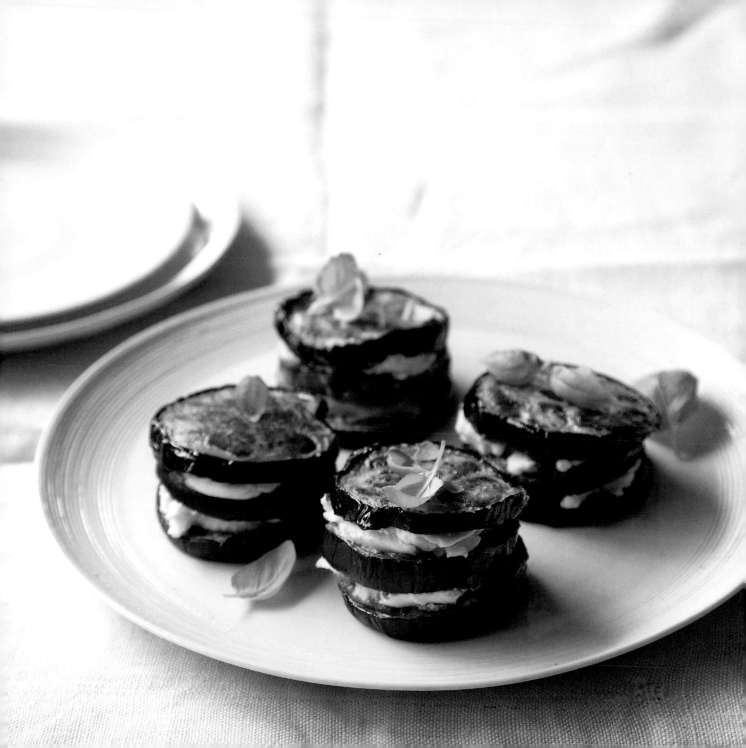

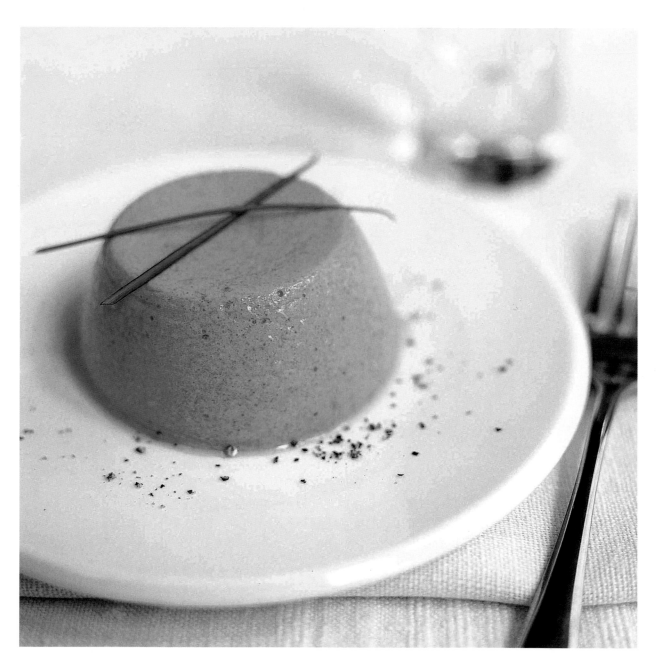

Red Pepper and Goat's Cheese Timbales

Very elegant, coral-coloured custards with a velvety texture, these can be eaten warm or cold with a small salad of young leaves. Team up with Avocado and Lemon Salad (see p.128) for an exquisite light lunch.

2 red peppers,
    about 325 g/11½ oz trimmed
    weight, halved and cored
300 g/11 oz mild, rindless soft
    goat's cheese
1 garlic clove, crushed with salt in
    a mortar or with a garlic crusher
2 organic eggs
Generous grinding of nutmeg
Butter, for greasing
Salt and freshly ground black pepper

Serves 4

Preheat the grill or oven to its highest setting. Place the peppers, cut side down, on a baking sheet and grill or roast until the skins are blackened and charred all over. Transfer to a plastic bag, tie the top, and leave to sweat until cool, then peel off the skins.

Preheat the oven to 150°C/300°F/Gas Mark 2. Place the roasted peppers, goat's cheese and garlic in a food processor and process until smooth. Season to taste. Add the eggs, one at a time, and a good grinding of nutmeg. Process until absolutely smooth.

Generously grease four ramekins with butter and place in a roasting tin or ovenproof dish. Divide the mixture among the ramekins. Pour boiling water into the roasting tin or dish to come halfway up the sides of the ramekins. Bake for 30 minutes, until firm. Remove from the oven and place the timbales on an oven rack to cool slightly, then turn out on to plates (to do this, place a plate upside down on top of each timbale and flip over). Remove the ramekin and serve.

Alternatively, leave to cool and serve chilled. To loosen from the ramekins, first stand in a bowl of hot water, then turn out.

Per serving
Carbs: 6 g protein: 21 g calories: 310 fibre: 1 g fat: 23 g (saturated fat: 14 g)

Field Mushrooms
with Blue Cheese Custard

These juicy little numbers will appreciate the company of a crisp lettuce salad such as cos and oak leaf dressed with a little salt, white wine vinegar and olive oil. Alternatively, turn them into a main course, paired up with Pumpkin and Swede Mash (see p.136).

6 large flat field or portobello
    mushrooms, about 340 g/12 oz,
    stems removed
2 tbsp olive oil
2 garlic cloves, chopped
Sea salt and freshly ground
    black pepper

For the blue cheese custard
75 g/3 oz blue cheese, such as
    Stilton, Roquefort or Gorgonzola,
    crumbled
150 ml/¼ pint crème fraîche
2 organic egg yolks
1 tbsp finely chopped fresh tarragon
    leaves, plus extra to garnish

Serves 6

Preheat the oven to 180°C/350°F/Gas Mark 4. Brush the mushroom caps with half the oil and place, gill side up, in an ovenproof dish just large enough to hold them in a single layer. Sprinkle the garlic over the gills, drizzle with the remaining oil and season with salt and pepper.

Beat together the cheese, crème fraîche, egg yolks and tarragon with a pinch of salt. Spoon the mixture into the mushroom caps. Bake for about 20 minutes, until the custard is set and bubbly and the mushrooms are soft. Sprinkle more chopped tarragon over the mushrooms and serve.

Per serving
Carbs: 1 g protein: 6 g calories: 207 fibre: 0.7 g fat: 20 g (saturated fat: 11 g)

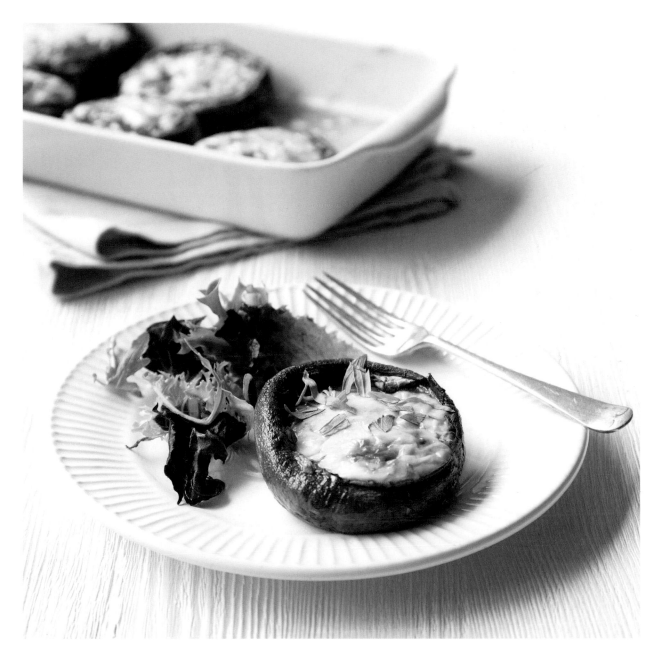

Halloumi-Stuffed Peppers

Here's one of my favourite ways to stuff peppers with no fuss. The recipe is very easy to multiply if you're feeding a crowd. These make a good partner for Roasted Aubergines with Dill Sauce (see p.133).

2 red peppers

4 basil leaves

1 large garlic clove, sliced

1 tbsp pine nuts

75 g/2½ oz halloumi cheese,
    cut into 4 slices or rough cubes
    (use feta if halloumi
    is unavailable)

4 tbsp olive oil

Serves 2, or 4 as an
accompaniment

Preheat the oven to 200°C/400°F/Gas Mark 6.

Cut the peppers in half from stem to base and de-seed but leave the stems intact. Place, skin side down, on a baking sheet. Place a basil leaf in each pepper half, sprinkle with garlic and pine nuts, top with a slice of halloumi and finish with a tablespoon of olive oil in each pepper half.

Bake for 20–30 minutes, until the cheese is golden.

Per serving
Carbs: 4 g protein: 4 g calories: 195 fibre: 1.25 g fat: 17 g (saturated fat: 4.5 g)

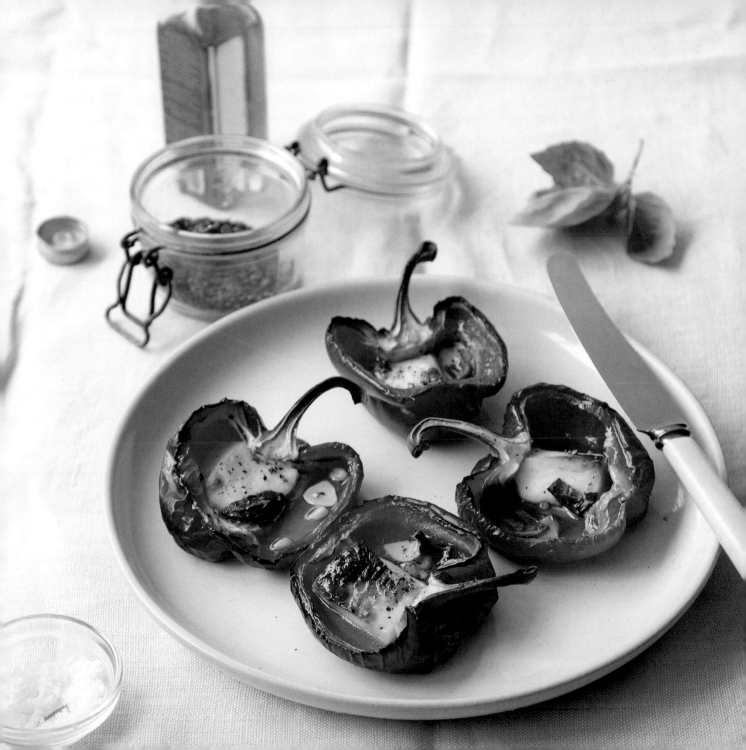

Aubergine Rarebit

This is a filling, warming taste of cheese heaven, with roasted aubergine rounds replacing the traditional toast.

1 large aubergine,
    sliced into 8 rounds
1 tbsp olive oil,
    plus extra for greasing
    and brushing
4 shallots or 1 medium onion,
    sliced
5 tbsp white wine
100 g/3½ oz grated Cheddar
    or other mature, tangy cheese
1 tsp dry mustard
2 organic eggs, beaten
Salt and freshly ground black pepper

Serves 4

Preheat the oven to 190°C/375°F/Gas Mark 5.

Brush each aubergine round all over with olive oil and place on a baking sheet lined with non-stick paper. Season with salt and pepper, and bake for 20–30 minutes, until softened and barely golden.

Preheat the grill to its highest setting. Alternatively, increase the oven temperature to 220°C/425°F/Gas Mark 7.

Heat a heavy pan over a medium heat, add the olive oil and cook the shallots or onion until softened. Turn the heat down as low as possible and add the wine, cheese and mustard to the pan, stirring until the cheese melts. Add the beaten eggs and stir until the mixture thickens slightly, but remove from the heat before the eggs scramble. Spoon the mixture on to the baked aubergines, and grill or bake until puffed and patched with gold. Grind over some black pepper and serve.

Per serving
Carbs: 3 g protein: 11 g calories: 200 fibre: 2 g fat: 15 g (saturated fat: 7 g)

Spiced Charred Aubergines

In this unusual cooking method, the aubergines steam in an aromatic broth which reduces to a thick glaze, and finally becomes a slightly charred crust. You will need a large, non-stick frying pan with a lid for this. Just remember – don't stir. Serve with salad or cooked spinach.

2 medium aubergines,
    about 600 g/1 lb 5 oz,
    cut into 2.5 cm/1 inch dice

2 tsp coriander seeds, lightly crushed

1 tsp cumin seeds

½ tsp ground turmeric

1 tsp salt, or to taste

1 large green chilli, cut into 3–4 pieces

Large handful of fresh coriander,
    chopped

Freshly ground black pepper

250 ml/8 fl oz water

50 g/2 oz butter, diced

Serves 4

Arrange the aubergines in an even layer in a large, non-stick frying pan. Sprinkle evenly with the coriander seeds, cumin seeds, turmeric, salt, chilli and chopped coriander, and season with pepper. Pour in the water and dot with butter. Cover the pan, place over a high heat and bring to the boil. Shake the pan a few times and lower the heat to a simmer. Cook, covered and without stirring, for about 20 minutes, checking occasionally that the water has not dried out – if it has, add a little more.

After 20 minutes, the aubergines should be buttery soft and the liquid should have reduced to a thick glaze. Do not stir. Remove the lid and increase the heat. Reduce the sauce until it just starts to form a crust on the base of the pan. Remove from the heat.

Leave to stand for 2 minutes, then stir the crust through the aubergines. Serve hot or cold.

Per serving
Carbs: 3.5 g protein: 1.5 g calories: 116 fibre: 3 g fat: 11 g (saturated fat: 7 g)

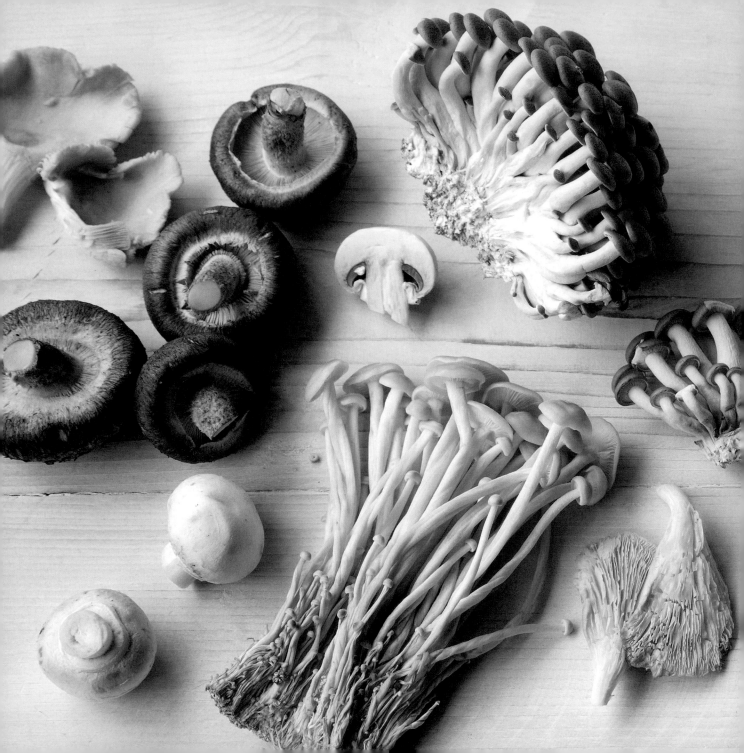

03: LIGHT LUNCH

Hearty soups and main-event salads feature here, perfect for a midday refuelling. Don't just restrict them to lunch – hot soups are perfect for winter nights, cool salads for balmy evenings...

Egg and Avocado Caesar

I call this "Caesar" because of the sharp, eggy dressing that gives it a resemblance to the classic salad. Avocado and olives make it a well-rounded and substantial lunch or supper.

6 organic eggs

4 tbsp freshly grated Parmesan cheese

4 tbsp white wine vinegar

1 tsp vegetarian Worcestershire sauce
    or light soy sauce

A small handful of fresh chives,
    snipped

Salt and freshly ground black pepper

4 tbsp olive oil

2 ripe avocados

Juice of ½ lemon

2 hearts of cos or romaine lettuce, torn

100 g/3½ oz good-quality black olives,
    such as Kalamata

Serves 4

Place the eggs in a small pan of cold water and bring to the boil. Boil for 7 minutes, then drain and rinse under cold water until cool. Crack and remove the shell and rinse again.

To make the dressing, place 2 shelled eggs in a bowl and mash well with a fork. Add the Parmesan, vinegar, Worcestershire or soy sauce and chives, season with salt and pepper and whisk thoroughly. Gradually whisk in the oil. (The dressing can also be whizzed with a hand blender or in a food processor if you want it completely smooth.)

Quarter the remaining eggs. Just before serving, peel, stone and quarter the avocados and sprinkle lightly with lemon juice to prevent discoloration. Make a bed of lettuce on each plate and top with avocados, egg quarters and olives. Spoon the dressing over the salad.

Per serving
Carbs: 2 g protein: 20 g calories: 480 fibre: 3.5 g fat: 43 g (saturated fat: 11 g)

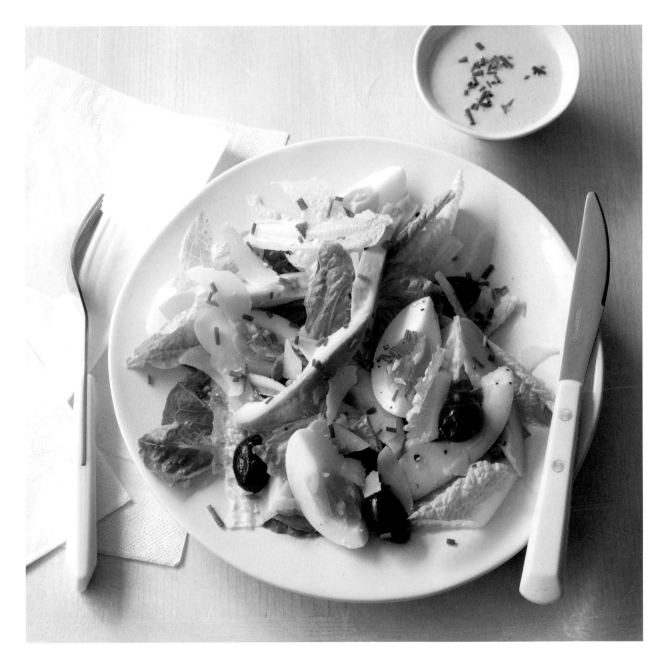

Curried Celeriac Soup with Coriander Oil

Thank heaven for celeriac, one of the few low-carb root vegetables. It gives this soup a creamy and satisfying texture. Ground almonds add richness and protein. Whole spices always produce the best flavour, but you can use ground spices instead if you're feeling lazy. The coriander oil is optional, but it makes the soup look and taste even more fabulous.

2 tsp coriander seeds
1 tsp cumin seeds
½ tsp chilli flakes, or to taste
25 g/1 oz/2 tbsp butter
2 tsp ground turmeric
1 large onion, chopped
3 garlic cloves, chopped
2.5 cm/1 inch piece of fresh
    root ginger, chopped
4 tbsp ground almonds
750 g/1 lb 10 oz celeriac, diced
1.2 litres/2 pints Vegetable Stock
    (see p.162)
Salt and freshly ground black pepper

For the coriander oil
1 small garlic clove
½ tsp coarse sea salt
Handful of coriander leaves
4 tbsp olive oil

4 tbsp double cream, to serve

Serves 6

To make the soup, grind together the coriander seeds, cumin seeds and chilli flakes in a spice grinder or pound in a mortar with a pestle. Melt the butter in a pan over a low heat. Add the crushed spices and the turmeric and cook for about 1 minute, until fragrant. Add the onion, cover and cook for about 5 minutes, until translucent. Add the garlic, ginger and almonds and cook for 1 minute. Add the celeriac and stock and bring to the boil. Simmer for 20 minutes, until the celeriac is tender, then purée the soup with a hand-held blender or food processor until smooth. Season to taste with salt and pepper.

To make the coriander oil, grind all the ingredients together in a spice grinder or food processor, or pound to a smooth paste in a mortar with a pestle.

To serve, ladle the soup into bowls and garnish with the coriander oil and cream. Sesame and Black Pepper Crispbreads (see p.108) are a good companion to this soup.

Per serving
Carbs: 6 g protein: 4.5 g calories: 237 fibre: 6 g fat: 21 g (saturated fat: 7 g)

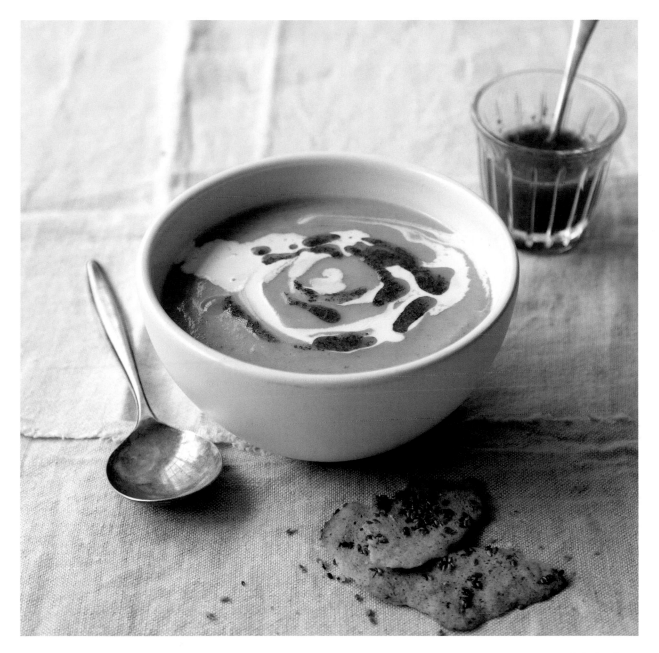

Cauliflower, Coconut and Cardamom Soup

A thick and substantial potage, where three C's come together to form a dazzling combo. Two equally appealing textures can be achieved with this soup – chunky or smooth.

1 tbsp sunflower oil
500 g/1¼ lb cauliflower, chopped
150 g/5 oz courgette, chopped
2 garlic cloves, chopped
3 spring onions (whites and clean greens), chopped
Sea salt and freshly ground black pepper
½ tsp cardamom seed (from about 20 pods), ground or pounded in a mortar or spice grinder
A good grinding of nutmeg
250 ml/½ pint coconut milk
375 ml/⅔ pint Vegetable Stock (see p.162)

Serves 4

Heat a lidded pot over a moderate flame and add oil. Add cauliflower, courgette, garlic and spring onion with a sprinkling of salt, pepper, the cardamom and nutmeg. Stir, cover and sweat for about 10 minutes, stirring from time to time.

Pour in the coconut milk and stock, and bring to the boil. Simmer for 10 minutes, or until the cauliflower is meltingly tender. Cool slightly, then for a slightly chunky texture, use a potato masher to crush the soup. Alternatively, use a hand-blender to purée until smooth.

Sesame and Black Pepper Crispbreads (see p.108) are a good companion to this soup.

Per serving
Carbs: 8 g protein: 8 g calories: 192 fibre: 3 g fat: 15 g (saturated fat: 6 g)

Chinese-Spice Tofu and Baby Leaf Salad

Tofu just needs a little loving attention to give it life. This simple treatment gives it masses of flavour, a light, crisp texture on the outside, and a creamy interior.

500 g/1¼ lb fresh firm tofu

4 tbsp sunflower oil

6 spring onions, sliced

4 garlic cloves, sliced

4 cm/1½ inch piece of fresh root ginger, grated

2 tsp Chinese five-spice powder

Salt

4 tbsp dark soy sauce

2 tbsp rice vinegar

2 tbsp sweetener

200 g/7 oz baby leaf salad

Serves 4

Drain the tofu and wrap in kitchen paper. Set aside while you prepare the remaining ingredients.

When you are ready to cook, cut the tofu into 2.5 cm/1 inch cubes. Heat the oil in a large, non-stick frying pan over a medium heat and add the tofu, spring onions, garlic, ginger, five-spice powder and a pinch of salt. Stir-fry for about 3 minutes, until the tofu is a light golden colour.

Add the soy sauce, vinegar and sweetener. Heat through, then remove the pan from the heat. Transfer the mixture to a bowl and leave to cool.

Toss the cooled tofu mixture through the baby leaves and serve immediately.

Per serving
Carbs: 3 g protein: 12 g calories: 210 fibre: 0.7 g fat: 17 g (saturated fat: 2 g)

Tofu, Mint and Palm Heart Salad with Hot and Spicy Dressing

Mint, ginger, garlic, chilli and toasted sesame seeds all sing a lovely harmony in this multi-textural, clean-flavoured salad. If palm hearts are not available, use canned water chestnuts.

250 g/9 oz fresh firm tofu, drained, patted dry, and cut into 2 cm/¾ inch cubes

1 quantity Sweet Chilli Sauce (see p.166), made with green chillies

2 tbsp sesame seeds

2 tsp sesame oil

8 Chinese cabbage leaves, lower halves shredded, top halves left intact

Small bunch of fresh mint, leaves stripped

1 x 400 g/14 oz can palm hearts, drained (225 g/8 oz drained weight), diagonally sliced

2.5 cm/1 inch piece of fresh root ginger, cut into slivers

Serves 4

Place the tofu in a shallow dish and pour the chilli sauce over it. Leave to marinate at room temperature for 30 minutes or for longer in the refrigerator.

Heat a dry frying pan over a medium heat and add sesame seeds. Cook, stirring occasionally, until golden and popping. Transfer to a small bowl and leave to cool.

Drain the tofu, reserving the sauce. Mix the sauce with the sesame oil, beating well.

To assemble the salad, arrange two Chinese cabbage leaf tops on each of four plates. Mix together the shredded leaves, mint, palm hearts and ginger slivers and divide among the plates. Top with marinated tofu and toasted sesame seeds. Spoon the dressing over each salad.

Per serving
Carbs: 4 g protein: 8.5 g calories: 135 fibre: 1 g fat: 8 g (saturated fat: 1 g)

Cyprus Salad

Resembling its sister the Greek salad (also a low-carb choice), this salad uses Cyprus's unique cheese, halloumi, instead of feta. If you can't find halloumi, try slicing feta in the same way and grilling until golden on top.

100 g/3½ oz broccoli florets

Half a cucumber, about 150 g/5 oz, chopped into chunks

3 celery sticks, chopped into chunks

1 green pepper, cored and chopped into chunks

1 red pepper, cored and chopped into chunks

50 g/2 oz good-quality black olives, such as Kalamata

Handful of fresh flat-leaf parsley, chopped

Handful of fresh mint leaves, chopped

250 g/9 oz halloumi cheese, sliced across the narrow end into 8 slices

Juice of ½ a lemon

For the dressing

½ small red onion, chopped

2 tbsp fresh lemon juice

1 tsp fresh or dried thyme

Sea salt and freshly ground black pepper

4 tbsp extra-virgin olive oil

Serves 4

First make the dressing. Mix together the onion, lemon juice and thyme, and season with sea salt and pepper. Whisk in the olive oil, then taste and adjust the seasoning if necessary. Set aside for the flavours to mingle while you prepare the rest of the salad.

Boil, microwave or steam the broccoli florets for 3 minutes, until just tender. Refresh under cold running water, drain and pat dry.

Mix together the broccoli, cucumber, celery, peppers, olives and herbs in a bowl.

When you are ready to serve, heat a large, non-stick frying pan over a medium heat. Do not add oil. Arrange the halloumi slices in the pan. Cook until golden underneath, then turn over and cook the other side. Meanwhile, stir the dressing through the salad and spoon onto plates.

As soon as the halloumi is golden, squeeze the lemon juice over it in the hot pan and remove from the heat. Place the halloumi on top of the salad and serve immediately.

Per serving
Carbs: 8 g protein: 12 g calories: 311 fibre: 3 g fat: 25 g (saturated fat: 10 g)

Warm Exotic Mushroom Salad

I was lucky enough to be asked to present a short film for UKTV Food about a mushroom farm in Kent in southeast England. The farmer, Nigel Baddeley, grows exotic varieties from Japan in England: shimeji, nameko and eringii mushrooms, which each have a unique, nutty flavour. I created this recipe with the produce he gave me, but you could use any combination of wild or cultivated types, especially shiitake and oyster mushrooms.

25 g/1 oz/2 tbsp butter
2 garlic cloves, chopped
300 g/11 oz mixed wild and
   cultivated mushrooms,
   sliced if large
1 tsp fresh thyme leaves
100 ml/3½ fl oz Madeira wine
75 g/3 oz mascarpone cheese
2 Little Gem lettuces
Sea salt and freshly ground
   black pepper

Serves 4

Melt the butter in a wide frying pan over a low heat and cook the garlic until fragrant. Add the mushrooms, season with salt and pepper and cook gently until softened. Add the thyme and Madeira, and cook for a further 2 minutes. Stir in mascarpone and cook until it coats the mushrooms. Remove the pan from the heat and cool briefly.

Arrange the lettuce leaves on plates and spoon the warm mushroom mixture over them. Serve immediately.

Per serving
Carbs: 1 g protein: 2 g calories: 171 fibre: 1 g fat: 14 g (saturated fat: 9 g)

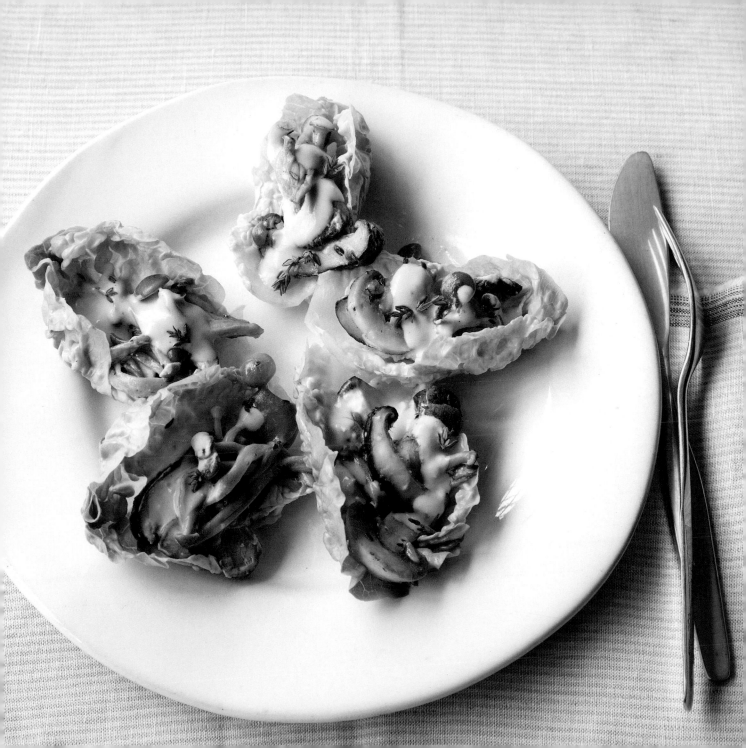

Warm Poached Egg Salad
with Tarragon Vinaigrette

My good friend Jennifer Joyce has kindly let me use this recipe from her gorgeous book *The Well-Dressed Salad*. This sophisticated salad is fully appreciated, she insists, "with a glass of chilled white Burgundy". I couldn't agree more – and only 1 g carbohydrate per glass!

4 organic eggs
200 g/7 oz green beans, trimmed
1 tbsp olive oil
Salt

For the dressing
2 tsp Dijon mustard
1 tsp red wine vinegar
½ tsp sea salt
Freshly ground black pepper
175 ml/6 fl oz olive oil
1 tbsp capers, rinsed and chopped
1 tbsp finely chopped flat-leaf parsley
Leaves from 2 tarragon sprigs,
    chopped
1 tbsp finely chopped shallot

Serves 4

First, poach the eggs. Bring a 2 cm/¾ inch depth of water to the boil in a large, non-stick frying pan. Reduce the heat to a low simmer. One at a time, carefully break each egg into a cup, then slide it into the water. Simmer for 2 minutes. Turn off the heat and let the eggs stand in the water for 10 minutes. They will then be perfectly cooked if you like the yolk slightly runny. If you prefer a well-done yolk, put the pan back on the heat for 1–2 minutes, until cooked to your liking. Place a couple of layers of kitchen paper on a plate. Remove the eggs from the pan with a slotted spatula and dry briefly on the paper. Keep warm if necessary.

Meanwhile, cook the beans and make the dressing. Bring a small pan of salted water to the boil. Blanch the beans for about 2 minutes, until tender but still firm. Drain and cool under cold running water or plunge into iced water to stop the cooking process.

To make the dressing, whisk together the mustard, vinegar, salt and pepper to taste in a small bowl. Gradually whisk in the oil to emulsify. Stir in the capers, herbs and shallot.

Return the beans to the dry pan and add the olive oil. Warm through over a medium heat. Place the warm beans on individual plates, top with an egg and spoon the dressing over them.

Per serving
Carbs: 4 g protein: 9 g calories: 436 fibre: 1.5 g fat: 42 g (saturated fat: 7 g)

Teriyaki Tofu
with Roasted Broccoli

Teriyaki is a rich and powerful Japanese flavour combination which brings out the best in tofu, and broccoli loves its company as well. Serve this with a few slices of cool cucumber to balance the salty-sweet flavour.

100 ml/3½ fl oz dark soy sauce

200 ml/7 fl oz dry sherry

1 cm/½ inch piece of fresh root ginger, finely grated

200 g/7 oz tofu, patted dry and cut into 2 triangles

4 tsp sunflower oil

200 g/7 oz broccoli florets

Cucumber slices, to serve (optional)

Serves 2

Preheat the oven to 200°C/400°F/Gas Mark 6. Place the soy sauce, sherry and ginger in a small frying pan and bring to the boil. Add the tofu and simmer for 5 minutes, then turn the tofu over and simmer for a further 5 minutes. Carefully lift the tofu from the sauce and place in a lightly oiled ovenproof dish. Reserve the sauce. Brush the top and sides of the tofu with 2 tsp oil.

Place the broccoli in a bowl and toss in the remaining oil. Arrange the broccoli around the tofu. Pour the reserved sauce over the broccoli and tofu. Roast for 25 minutes, until the broccoli is cooked and slightly crisp. Serve hot with cucumber slices, if you like.

Per serving
Carbs: 1.7g protein: 7 g calories: 116 fibre: 2 g fat: 9 g (saturated fat: 1 g)

Spanish Tortilla
with Courgettes and Manchego

Choose a smallish, reliable non-stick pan for the tortilla, with a heatproof handle that will be safe under the grill, ideally about 25 cm/10 inches in diameter. This may seem too small for the initial frying of the courgettes, but they do shrink considerably.

750 g/1 lb 10 oz courgettes,
    thinly sliced
2 tbsp olive oil
3 organic eggs
Sea salt and freshly ground
    black pepper
100 g/3 ½ oz Manchego, feta,
    or other tangy cheese,
    cut into small dice

Serves 6

Heat a small, non-stick frying pan over a medium heat and add 1 tbsp olive oil. Add the courgettes, season with a little salt and pepper, and cook, moving them around frequently, until soft and golden.

Preheat the grill to its highest setting. Break the eggs into a large bowl and beat well with a little salt and pepper. Stir the courgettes and cheese into the eggs until the courgettes are well coated.

Return the pan to the heat and add the remaining olive oil. Scoop the egg mixture into the pan.

Cook, loosening the edges occasionally, until the tortilla is deep golden underneath and loose when you shake the pan. Place the pan under the grill and cook until the egg is set throughout and the top is patched with gold. Carefully remove the tortilla from the pan and cool. Serve warm or cold, cut into wedges.

Per serving
Carbs: 2.5 g protein: 10 g calories: 187 fibre: 1 g fat: 15 g (saturated fat: 5 g)

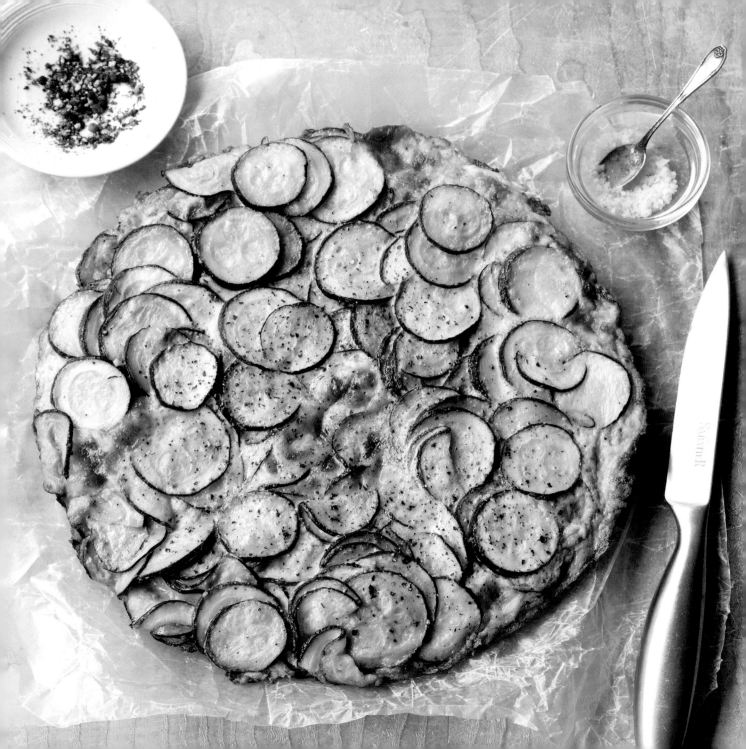

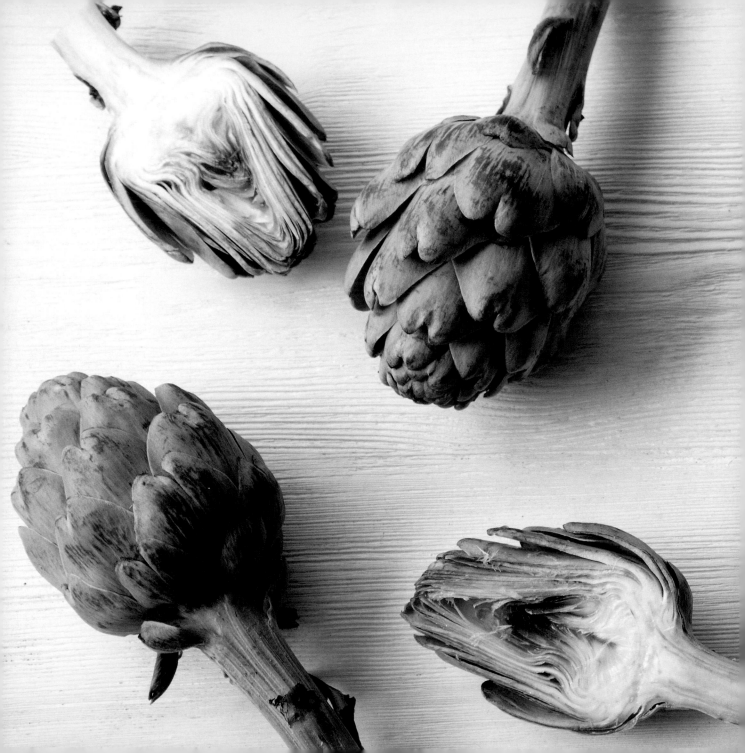

04:
MAIN
COURSES

Feed your friends and family with these substantial dishes – tarts, gratins, stews, curries and comfort food. Even those not on a low-carb diet can't fail to feel satisfied.

Vietnamese Asparagus Pancakes

This coconut batter is something that I dreamed up, but it fits deliciously into a Vietnamese-style pancake platter, with the essential cucumber and herb salad and hot-sweet sauce. If asparagus is out of season, try using lightly stir-fried beansprouts instead, or simply fill the pancakes with cucumber batons, coriander and mint sprigs.

2 bunches asparagus,
    about 250 g/9 oz total
4 tsp sunflower oil
4 spring onions, sliced

For the batter
4 tbsp soy flour
3 organic eggs
100 ml/3½ fl oz canned coconut milk
½ tsp ground turmeric
Large pinch of salt

To serve
½ cucumber, about 150 g/5 oz, cut
    into batons or sliced
4 fresh coriander sprigs
4 fresh mint sprigs
1 quantity Sweet Chilli Sauce
    (see p.166)

Serves 4

Preheat the oven to 120°C/250°F/Gas Mark ½ for keeping warm. Steam the asparagus in a pan or in the microwave for 3 minutes, or until cooked to your liking. Keep warm.

To make the batter, place the flour, eggs, coconut milk, turmeric and salt in a blender and process until smooth. Heat a medium, non-stick frying pan over a medium heat and add 1 tsp oil. Pour in a quarter of the batter in a thin layer and swirl the pan to coat the base. Sprinkle with a quarter of the spring onions before it sets. When golden underneath, flip the pancake over and cook until golden on the other side. Transfer to a plate and keep warm. Make three more pancakes in the same way, adding 1 tsp oil to the pan each time.

To serve, roll a pancake around a bundle of asparagus, starting from the edge. Serve with cucumber, coriander and mint sprigs and a small bowl of sweet chilli sauce.

Per serving
Carbs: 7 g protein: 14 g calories: 230 fibre: 3.6 g fat: 16 g (saturated fat: 2 g)

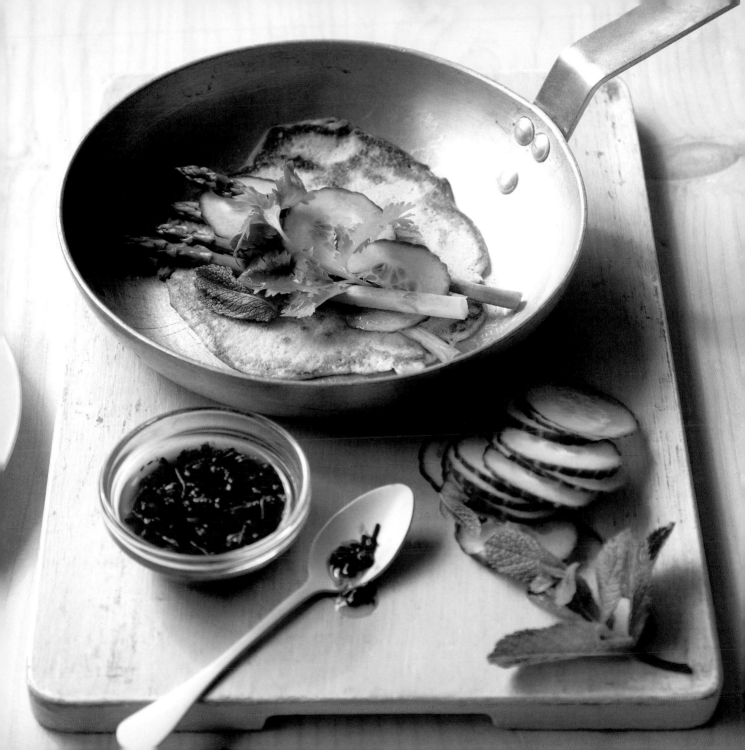

Rocket and Ricotta Cheesecake

A creamy, savoury cheesecake, lightened with rocket and herbs. Serve with a crunchy leaf salad, or for a more full-on meal, with Braised Fennel and Peppers (see p.132).

Butter, for greasing
75 g/3 oz walnut pieces
1 tbsp olive oil
3 garlic cloves, chopped
3 spring onions, chopped
200 g/7 oz rocket, coarsely chopped
3 tbsp chopped fresh herbs,
    such as parsley, basil and dill,
    plus extra to garnish
3 organic eggs
500 g/1¼ lb ricotta cheese, drained
4 tbsp freshly grated Parmesan
    cheese, plus extra shavings
    to garnish
Sea salt and freshly ground
    black pepper

Serves 6

Preheat the oven to 160°C/325°F/Gas Mark 3. Generously butter a 20 cm/8 inch cake tin with a loose base. Grind the walnut pieces to a powder in a food processor, then press them into the base and sides of the tin.

Heat a frying pan over a low heat and add the olive oil. Cook the garlic and spring onions for 1 minute, until fragrant. Add the rocket and herbs and stir for 1–2 minutes, until the rocket is just wilted. Remove the pan from the heat.

Put the eggs, ricotta, Parmesan and the rocket mixture in a clean food processor, and season with salt and pepper. Process until evenly mixed. Pour into the prepared tin. Bake for about 45 minutes, until golden and firm. Turn out, cut into wedges and serve warm.

Per serving
Carbs: 3 g protein: 15 g calories: 293 fibre: 0.8 g fat: 24 g (saturated fat: 9 g)

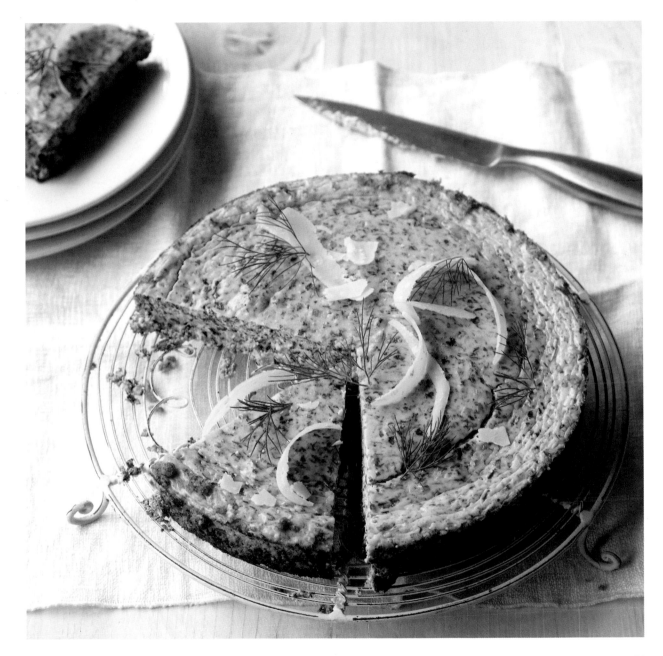

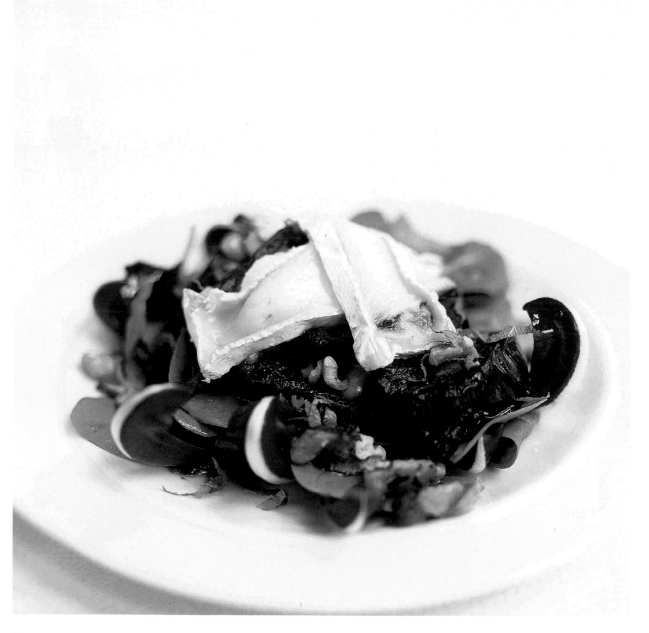

Warm Salad of Aubergines and Melting Camembert

Get ready for some guilt-free indulgence with this upmarket salad. Salting the aubergines will prevent them from absorbing too much oil.

2 medium aubergines,
    sliced into 1 cm/½ inch rounds
Olive oil
4 shallots, sliced
100 ml/3½ fl oz dry vermouth
    or white wine
1 tbsp wine vinegar
2 radicchio or treviso, leaves torn
125 g/4½ oz young spinach leaves
200 g/7 oz chilled Camembert cheese,
    sliced into strips
50 g/2 oz walnuts, lightly crushed
Handful of fresh mint leaves, chopped
Salt and freshly ground black pepper

Serves 4

Spread out the aubergine rounds in a colander and sprinkle with salt. Leave to drain for 30 minutes over the sink, then pat dry.

Heat a large frying pan over a medium heat and add 4 tbsp olive oil. Cook the aubergines, in batches if necessary, until soft and golden, adding a little more oil if necessary. Remove the aubergines and add a drop more oil to the pan, then cook the shallots until soft. Return all the aubergines to the pan and reheat.

Add the vermouth or wine all at once – stand back as it may splutter at first. Season well with salt and pepper and cook, shaking the pan gently, until the liquid has reduced by half. Add the vinegar to the pan and shake. Cook for a further 2 minutes, while the juices thicken and caramelise, then remove the pan from the heat. Preheat the grill to its highest setting.

Meanwhile, make a bed of radicchio and young spinach leaves on a heatproof platter. Top with the aubergines and pan juices. Place slices of Camembert on the summit. Sprinkle with walnuts. Place the platter under the grill until the cheese starts to melt. Finally, sprinkle with chopped mint and serve.

Per serving
Carbs: 5 g protein: 1 g calories: 162 fibre: 2 g fat: 13 g (saturated fat: 2 g)

Creamy Celeriac Gratin

This makes a generous quantity, and believe me, you are going to want leftovers!
It also freezes well. Serve with Ruby Chard with Pine Nuts and Redcurrants (see p.131).

Butter, for greasing

3 garlic cloves

1 tsp coarse salt

1 large celeriac, 700 g/1½ lb trimmed
    weight, peeled and grated

Generous grinding of nutmeg

300 ml/½ pint double cream

50 g/2 oz ground almonds

2 tbsp chopped fresh parsley

4 tbsp freshly grated Parmesan cheese

Salt and freshly ground black pepper

Serves 8

Preheat the oven to 200°C/400°F/Gas Mark 6. Lightly grease a gratin dish.

Crush the garlic in a mortar with the salt until smooth (alternatively use a garlic crusher).

Mix together the salted garlic, celeriac, nutmeg and cream in a large bowl and season with pepper. Stir until well mixed – it helps to use clean hands to combine the mixture thoroughly. Spoon the mixture into the gratin dish and pack down.

Mix together the almonds, parsley and Parmesan. Sprinkle over the top of the gratin. Bake for about 40 minutes, until soft and golden.

Per serving
Carbs: 3 g protein: 6 g calories: 271 fibre: 4 g fat: 26 g (saturated fat: 14 g)

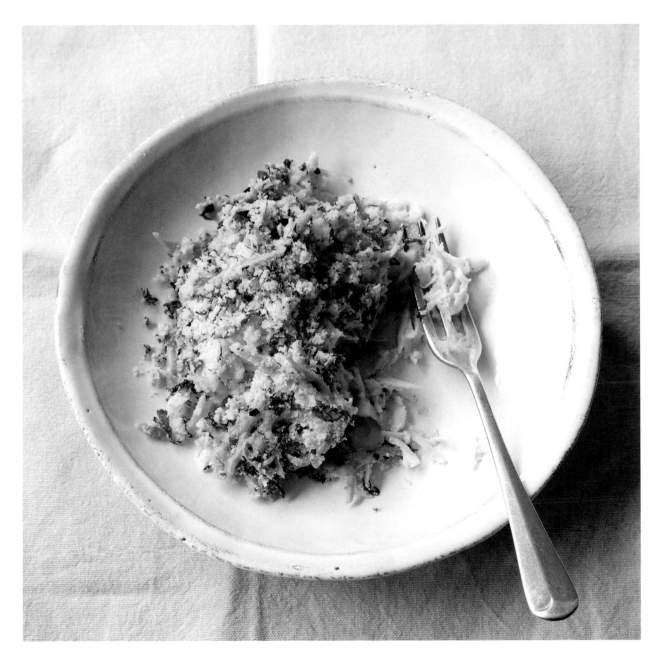

Thai Hot and Sour Salad with Crispy Tofu

Here's a user-friendly version of the classic Thai salad "som tam". Low-carb swede takes the place of green papaya and the tofu bumps up the protein quotient.

200 g/7 oz firm tofu
Sunflower oil, for frying

For the dressing

2 red chillies, de-seeded if large
2 garlic cloves
4 tbsp light soy sauce
4 tbsp lime juice
4 tbsp sweetener

For the salad

300 g/11 oz swede, grated
100 g/3½ oz green beans,
　　sliced lengthways
1 red pepper, cored and thinly sliced
4 spring onions, sliced
2 handfuls of fresh mint leaves
50 g/2 oz toasted peanuts, ground

Serves 4

First, drain the tofu and wrap in kitchen paper until ready to use.

Make the dressing by pounding all the ingredients in a heavy mortar or by processing them in a blender. Combine the swede, beans, pepper, spring onions, mint, and half the peanuts. Stir half the dressing through the salad.

Heat a shallow layer of oil in a frying pan over a high heat. Cut the tofu into 7.5 cm/3 inch slices and fry, turning once, until golden all over. Drain on kitchen paper.

Spoon the salad on to plates and top with the tofu. Finish with the remaining dressing and sprinkle with the remaining peanuts.

Per serving
Carbs: 10 g protein: 10 g calories: 159 fibre: 3.5 g fat: 9 g (saturated fat: 1.5 g)

Spinach and Ricotta Gnocchi with Sage Butter

These rich, yet fluffy gnocchi are a proper Italian luxury meal. They can also be placed in an ovenproof dish after boiling, covered in grated cheese and baked for a fabulous gratin.

200 g/7 oz young spinach, washed

2 tbsp chopped parsley

1 garlic clove, crushed

150 g/5 oz ricotta cheese, drained

75 g/3 oz soy flour

1 organic egg, plus 1 yolk

100 g/3½ oz freshly grated Parmesan cheese, plus extra to serve

Generous grating of nutmeg

Salt and freshly ground black pepper

For the sage butter

75 g/3 oz/6 tbsp unsalted butter

Pinch of salt

16 fresh sage leaves, coarsely chopped

Serves 4

Place the spinach in a bowl and pour boiling water over it. When it has wilted, drain and leave to cool. Wrap a clean tea towel around the spinach and, holding it over the sink, squeeze out as much moisture as possible. Chop finely.

Combine the chopped spinach with the parsley, garlic, ricotta, soy flour, egg and egg yolk, Parmesan and nutmeg. Season with salt and pepper. Stir vigorously until thoroughly combined.

Bring a large pan of water to the boil and salt it well. Form the dough into balls, about the size of a large cherry. (The gnocchi can be frozen at this stage if you're planning a future meal.) Drop a few gnocchi at a time into the water, lower the heat to a simmer and cook for 3–4 minutes, until they have risen to the surface. Remove with a slotted spoon. Keep warm while you cook the remaining gnocchi.

To make the sage butter, melt the butter in a pan over a medium heat. Add a pinch of salt and the sage. Cook until the sage is tinged with gold. Pour the herb butter over the cooked gnocchi and serve.

Per serving

Carbs: 6 g protein: 22 g calories: 409 fibre: 3 g fat: 33 g (saturated fat: 18 g)

Spaghetti Squash with Smoked Chilli Pesto

Some purists might say "Don't mess with pesto", but trust me, this combination works (see also Smoky Aubergine Timbales, p.42). The noodle-like squash, with its low-key flavour, is a perfect partner for this assertive pesto. Alternatively, serve with carb-free noodles or rice, available online and from speciality shops.

Olive oil
1 large spaghetti squash,
    about 750 g/1 lb 10 oz
25 g/1 oz freshly grated Parmesan
    cheese (optional)

For the smoked chilli pesto
1 dried smoked chilli,
    such as chipotle (optional)
2 tsp smoked paprika
Large bunch of basil
100 g/3½ oz pine nuts
2 garlic cloves, roughly chopped
50 g /2 oz freshly grated
    Parmesan cheese
½ tsp sea salt, or to taste
6 tbsp olive oil

Serves 4

Preheat the oven to 200°C/400°F/Gas Mark 6. Lightly oil a baking sheet. Cut the spaghetti squash in half from stem to base and scoop out the seeds and surrounding fibres. Place cut side down on the baking sheet and cook for 45–60 minutes, or until a skewer or fork pushed through the skin meets no resistance underneath. Leave until cool enough to handle. Leave the oven turned on.

Meanwhile, make the pesto. If using the dried chilli, place it in a small pan with boiling water and simmer for 15–20 minutes, until soft and rehydrated. Cool, de-seed and chop. Place the remaining pesto ingredients, except the olive oil, in a food processor with the chopped chilli and process until finely chopped. With the motor running, gradually add the oil until a thick paste forms.

Use a fork to pull all the spaghetti-like strands of squash away from the skin. Place in a bowl and toss with the pesto – if it seems difficult to distribute, a little splash of boiling water will help. Spoon into an ovenproof dish, sprinkle with the Parmesan, if using, and bake for 10–15 minutes, until heated through. Alternatively, simply reheat in a microwave until piping hot throughout and finish with grated Parmesan.

Per serving
Carbs: 10 g protein: 13 g calories: 462 fibre: 5 g fat: 41 g (saturated fat: 8 g)

Paneer Masala
with Spinach and Coconut

I've borrowed techniques from various regions of India's vast and varied cuisine for this quick stir-fry dish. The result may not be authentic, but it is certainly an exciting combination, and amazingly simple to prepare. Use store-bought paneer or discover how easy it is to make from scratch on p.163.

2 tbsp sunflower oil

1 tsp black mustard seeds

1 tsp cumin seeds

1 tsp ground turmeric

2 red chillies, slit

3 spring onions, sliced

3 garlic cloves, sliced

2.5 cm/1 inch piece of fresh root
    ginger, chopped

50 g/2 oz desiccated coconut

300 g/11 oz paneer, diced

200 g/7 oz young spinach, chopped

100 ml/3½ fl oz Greek yogurt

Serves 4

Heat a wok until moderately hot. Add the oil and mustard seeds. When the seeds pop, add the cumin, turmeric, chillies, spring onions, garlic and ginger, and cook for about 2 minutes, until golden and fragrant. Add the coconut and paneer, and cook until the paneer becomes light golden in colour.

Stir the spinach through the mixture and, as soon as it is completely wilted, remove the wok from the heat. Stir in the yogurt and serve hot.

Per serving
Carbs: 5 g protein: 12 g calories: 236 fibre: 3 g fat: 18 g (saturated fat: 10 g)

Tomato and Artichoke Stew

Canned or bottled artichoke hearts are a great convenience food and make this a sumptuous yet user-friendly dish. I originally made this dish using four large fresh artichoke hearts. Do try it with fresh if you're feeling up to the rather hairy process of removing all the leaves and the choke, then simmer in the sauce until tender.

3 tbsp olive oil

4 garlic cloves, crushed with
    1 tsp coarse salt in a mortar
    or with a garlic crusher

2 x 400 g/14 oz cans tomatoes,
    chopped

300 g/11 oz canned or bottled
    artichoke hearts, drained
    and halved if whole

1 tbsp red wine vinegar

2 tbsp chopped fresh flat-leaf
    parsley, plus extra to garnish

Pinch of dried chilli flakes

Sea salt and freshly ground
    black pepper

4 organic eggs

4–5 tbsp ricotta cheese

Serves 4

Heat the oil in a large pan. Add the garlic and cook, stirring. As soon as it becomes fragrant, add the tomatoes and artichokes. Bring to the boil, then add the vinegar, parsley and chilli. Season to taste with salt, if necessary, and pepper. Cover and simmer gently, stirring occasionally, for 10 minutes, then remove the lid and simmer for a further 10 minutes, until thickened.

Make four hollows with a spoon around the edge of the pan and break the eggs into them. Spoon ricotta in between the eggs. Cover the pan while the eggs cook. As soon as they are poached to your liking, serve the stew.

Per serving
Carbs: 8 g protein: 13 g calories: 233 fibre: 1.5 g fat: 17 g (saturated fat: 4 g)

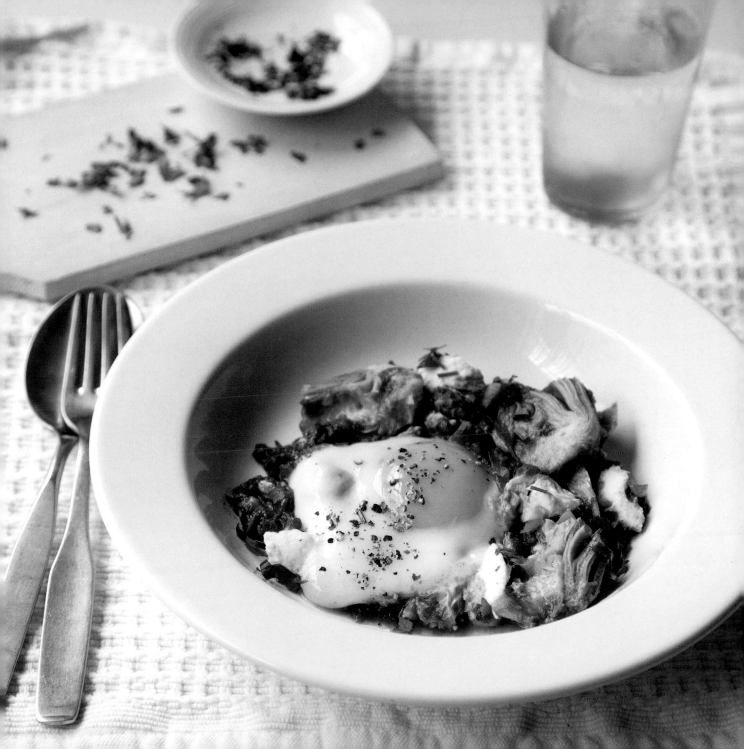

Tunisian Spiced Torte

This delicious crustless mint-flavoured quiche is inspired by a recipe from Tunisia called "Makhouda nahna".
I first came across it in the book *North Africa – The Vegetarian Table* by Kitty Morse. The torte keeps for days in
the refrigerator and is extremely portable, making it perfect for a picnic. Use dried mint from a herbal teabag
rather than a jar or packet – it tastes fresher and stronger.

Butter, for greasing

2 tbsp olive oil

2 onions, chopped

10 organic eggs

100 g/3½ oz ground almonds

Generous handful of fresh parsley,
    chopped

1 tbsp dried mint

1 tbsp mild smoked paprika/pimentón

250 g/9 oz Gruyère, or other mature,
    tangy cheese, diced

½ tsp salt

Freshly ground black pepper

Serves 8

Preheat the oven to 200°C/400°F/Gas Mark 6. Generously grease a 24 cm/9 inch
springform cake tin.

Heat the olive oil over a medium heat and cook the onions until lightly browned.

Beat the eggs in a large bowl, then stir in all remaining ingredients and add the
onions. Stir until thoroughly mixed. Pour the mixture into the prepared tin and bake
for 35–40 minutes, until a knife inserted in the middle comes out clean.

Leave to cool slightly, then run a sharp knife around the edge, unmould, and serve warm
or at room temperature.

Per serving
Carbs: 3 g protein: 21 g calories: 345 fibre: 1 g fat: 28 g (saturated fat: 10 g)

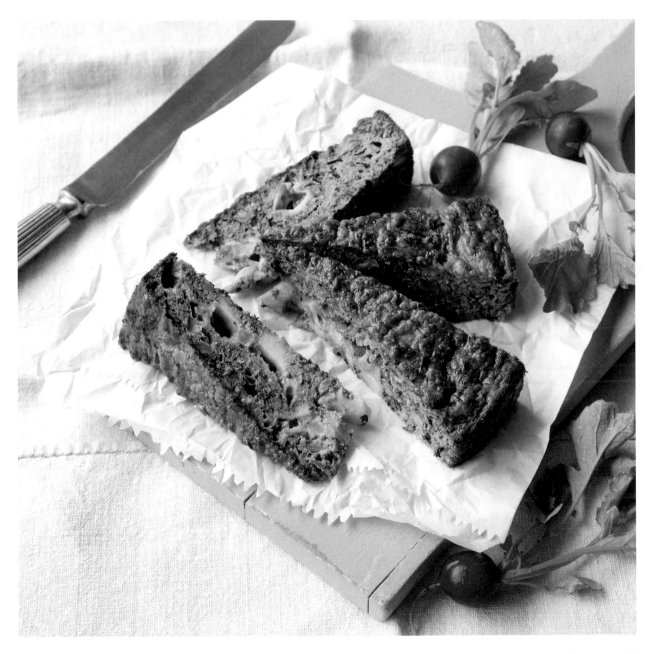

Egg Foo Yung

I consulted Norman Fu, Chef Lecturer in Chinese Cookery, to find out the secret of this classic Anglo-Chinese dish. It requires a smart trick (outlined below) to cook it to perfection – not too leaky and not too solid. Also, the eggs are cooked over a medium-low heat, because as Norman insists, "A good *foo yung* does not have any brown bits." No spices or sauces are used, because they just mask the delicate flavours of the dish.

2½ tbsp sunflower oil

3 tbsp chopped red pepper

3 tbsp chopped celery

3 tbsp chopped courgette

25 g/1 oz beansprouts

3 spring onions, sliced

4 organic eggs

Sea salt

Serves 2

Line a small colander with kitchen paper. Heat a well-seasoned wok or non-stick frying pan over a high heat and add 1 tsp of the oil. Add the pepper, celery, courgette, beansprouts, spring onions and a pinch of salt, and stir-fry for 1–2 minutes, until softened. Transfer the contents of the pan to the lined colander and leave to cool and drain. This ensures that the egg will not be diluted with cooking juices.

Beat the eggs with a little salt until mixed but not frothy. Stir in the cooled vegetables and mix well. Heat the wok or pan over a low to medium heat and add the remaining oil. Pour in the egg mixture and swirl in the pan. Push the mixture away from you while tilting the pan towards you, rather than scrambling vigorously, so the mixture runs gently on to the exposed areas. Repeat this action all over the pan until the egg is just set. Turn the whole *foo yung* over once, then slide on to a plate and serve immediately.

Per serving
Carbs: 3.5 g protein: 16 g calories: 293 fibre: 1 g fat: 25 g (saturated fat: 5 g)

Cabbage Gratin

Here, the modest cabbage gets dressed to the nines in a creamy golden crust, studded with caraway and lifted with the flavour of orange zest. Serve with steamed green beans.

1 tbsp olive oil

3 garlic cloves, chopped

600 g/1 lb 5 oz Savoy cabbage,
    trimmed weight, shredded

400 ml/14 fl oz reduced-fat crème
    fraîche or sour cream

3 organic egg yolks

50 g/2 oz grated Cheddar cheese

Finely grated zest of 1 orange

Several fresh thyme sprigs,
    leaves stripped

1 tsp caraway seeds

Salt and freshly ground black pepper

Serves 4

Heat the oil in a pan and cook the garlic until light golden. Add the cabbage and season well. Cover and cook, stirring frequently, for about 15 minutes, until the cabbage is tender.

Preheat the oven to 200°C/400°F/Gas Mark 6. Remove the pan from the heat. If there is liquid in the pan, drain it off. Spoon the cabbage into an ovenproof dish and pack down.

To make the custard, beat together the crème fraîche, egg yolks, Cheddar, orange rind and thyme leaves with a pinch of salt. Pour the mixture over the cabbage and sprinkle with the caraway seeds. Bake for 30–40 minutes, until the top is golden and bubbling around the edges.

Per serving

Carbs: 10 g protein: 10 g calories: 323 fibre: 3.5 g fat: 26 g (saturated fat: 14 g)

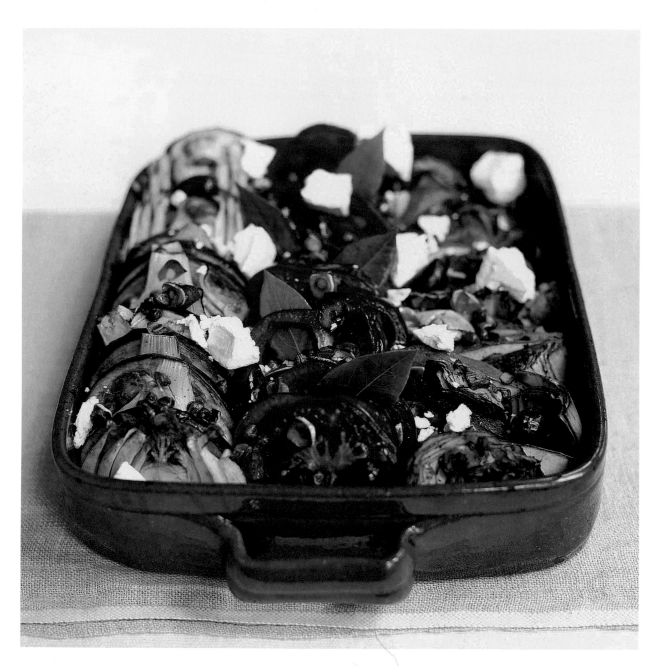

Provençal Tian

The arrangement of the vegetables in three colourful stripes makes this a *pièce de résistance*, although you can just throw it all in haphazardly without affecting the flavour. The recipe makes a generous quantity – leftovers are lovely to eat cold as a salad.

Butter, for greasing

1 red pepper, cored and sliced
    into rings

350 g/12 oz vine or plum tomatoes,
    sliced

350 g/12 oz courgettes,
    sliced in 1 cm/½ inch rounds

400 g/14 oz artichoke hearts,
    drained and halved

350 g/12 oz aubergine,
    sliced in 5 mm/¼ inch rounds

300 g/11 oz fennel, sliced

50 g /2 oz good-quality black olives

4 bay leaves

200 g/7 oz fresh goat's or feta cheese
    (optional)

Freshly ground black pepper

For the dressing

4 tbsp olive oil

1 tbsp balsamic vinegar

4 garlic cloves, thinly sliced

A handful of fresh basil, shredded

2 tbsp capers

1 tsp salt, or to taste

Serves 8

Preheat the oven to 200°C/400°F/Gas Mark 6. Lightly grease a wide rectangular ovenproof dish. Aim to interleave each pair of vegetables with one another: place the red bell pepper and tomatoes alternately in one red stripe across the top of the dish and the courgette and artichoke hearts in one green stripe across the bottom. Arrange the slices of aubergine and fennel in the middle.

Whisk together all the dressing ingredients and spoon almost all the mixture over the vegetables as evenly as possible. Brush every exposed surface with the remaining dressing. Season with plenty of pepper and garnish with olives and bay leaves.

Roast for 45–50 minutes, until the vegetables are soft, sizzling and well browned around the edges. Remove from the oven and crumble the goat's or feta cheese, if using, over the surface. Serve warm or cold.

Per serving

Carbs: 6 g protein: 9 g calories: 180 fibre: 3 g fat: 13 g (saturated fat: 6 g)

Luxury Cauliflower Cheese

Here's my variation on the classic comfort food, best served with a very simply dressed salad of crunchy leaves.

2 large trimmed leeks,
about 300 g/11 oz
1 large cauliflower,
about 500 g/1¼ lb,
broken into florets
1 tsp sea salt
2 bay leaves
300 ml/½ pint water
200 g/7 oz cream cheese
100 g/3½ oz grated Cheddar cheese
4 tbsp freshly grated Parmesan cheese
½ tsp dried chilli flakes, or to taste

Serves 4

Preheat the oven to 220°C/425°F/Gas Mark 7. Slice the leeks quite thickly and wash well, making sure no dirt is concealed in the upper parts. Place the leeks in a large pan with a lid. Place the cauliflower florets on top. Add the salt and bay leaves and pour in the water. Cover and bring to the boil over a high heat. Lower the heat and simmer for 5 minutes.

Remove the cauliflower, leeks and bay leaves from the pan and reserve the cooking liquid. Place the vegetables in a wide roasting tin or gratin dish in a snug single layer. Put the dish of vegetables in the oven to dry out while you prepare the cheese sauce.

Bring the reserved cooking liquid to the boil. Add the cream cheese, breaking it up with a whisk. Whisk until smooth and melted. Add the grated cheese and whisk until melted and thick, then remove from the heat.

Remove the vegetables from the oven and pour the cheese sauce evenly over them. Sprinkle the grated Parmesan over the top and dust with chilli flakes. Return to the oven and bake for about 20–30 minutes, until golden brown and bubbly.

Per serving
Carbs: 6 g protein: 18 g calories: 422 fibre: 4 g fat: 36 g (saturated fat: 22 g)

Cauliflower Mash
and Porcini Gravy for Sausages

The vegetarian sausages available nowadays get better and better as food technology improves. Many are soy-protein based and low-carb, but do check the label. Pan-fried halloumi cheese slices also make an excellent accompaniment to the mash and gravy.

For the mash
600 g/1 lb 5 oz cauliflower,
    trimmed weight
½ tsp salt
1 tbsp olive oil
Generous grinding of nutmeg

For the gravy
10 g/¼ oz dried porcini mushrooms
250 ml/8 fl oz boiling water
2 tbsp olive oil
1 leek, chopped
Leaves stripped from 2 fresh
    thyme sprigs
1 bay leaf
120 ml/4 fl oz dry vermouth
    or white wine
1 tbsp cornflour/cornstarch, mixed
    with 1 tbsp cold water
Sea salt and freshly ground
    black pepper
Low-carb vegetarian sausages

Serves 4

First, make the gravy. Place the porcini mushrooms in a bowl and pour the boiling water over them. Leave to soak for about 20 minutes. Fish the softened mushrooms out of the liquid, squeezing out excess moisture. Chop and set aside, reserving the soaking liquid.

Heat a frying pan over a medium heat and add the oil. Add the chopped leek and porcini and cook for about 3 minutes, until the leek is softened. Add the herbs and vermouth or wine. Pour the reserved mushroom soaking water through a fine sieve into the pan and season with salt and pepper. Bring to the boil. Stir in the cornflour mixed with water and cook, stirring, until thickened. Simmer gently for a few more minutes to thicken further and to evaporate the alcohol.

To make the mash, chop the cauliflower into fairly small pieces. Place in a heavy pan with the salt and oil, and stir. Cover and place over a medium heat until steaming, then lower the heat to a gentle simmer. Let the cauliflower cook in its own juice for 15–20 minutes, until very soft and collapsed. Remove the lid and let any remaining juices evaporate. Grind or grate in a generous dose of nutmeg, then mash until smooth. If it still seems too wet, continue steaming over the heat, stirring frequently.

Cook the vegetarian sausages according to the manufacturer's instructions. Serve the mash with the sausages and porcini gravy poured over the top.

Per serving
Carbs: 10 g protein: 6 g calories: 177 fibre: 3 g fat: 10 g (saturated fat: 2 g)

Paneer and Herb Fritters

A few of these delectable, crunchy little cakes make a satisfying meal with salad or green vegetables. Alternatively, make tiny fritters for party nibbles. You can use store-bought paneer, or make your own using the recipe on p.163.

250 g/9 oz paneer, grated or crumbled
50 g/2 oz fresh coriander sprigs
    and mint leaves, chopped
2.5 cm/1 inch piece of fresh root
    ginger, finely grated
2 garlic cloves, crushed
1 tsp coriander seeds, crushed,
    or 1 tsp ground coriander
1 tsp salt
2 organic eggs
2 tbsp soy flour
Sunflower oil, for frying
Freshly ground black pepper
Lemon wedges, to serve
1 quantity Sweet Chilli Sauce (p.166),
    to serve

Serves 4

Combine the paneer, herbs, ginger, garlic, coriander seeds, salt, eggs and flour in a bowl, season with pepper and mix very thoroughly. Using wet hands, take walnut-sized handfuls of the mixture, then squeeze and press into little flat patties. Set aside on a plate while you make all the cakes. Chill in the refrigerator until ready to cook.

Heat a shallow layer of oil in a non-stick pan over a medium heat. When hot, add the patties to the oil and cook until golden, then turn over and cook until completely golden. Drain on kitchen paper. Serve with lemon wedges to squeeze over them, and Sweet Chilli Sauce, if desired.

Per serving
Carbs: 4 g protein: 14 g calories: 165 fibre: 1 g fat: 10 g (saturated fat: 3 g)

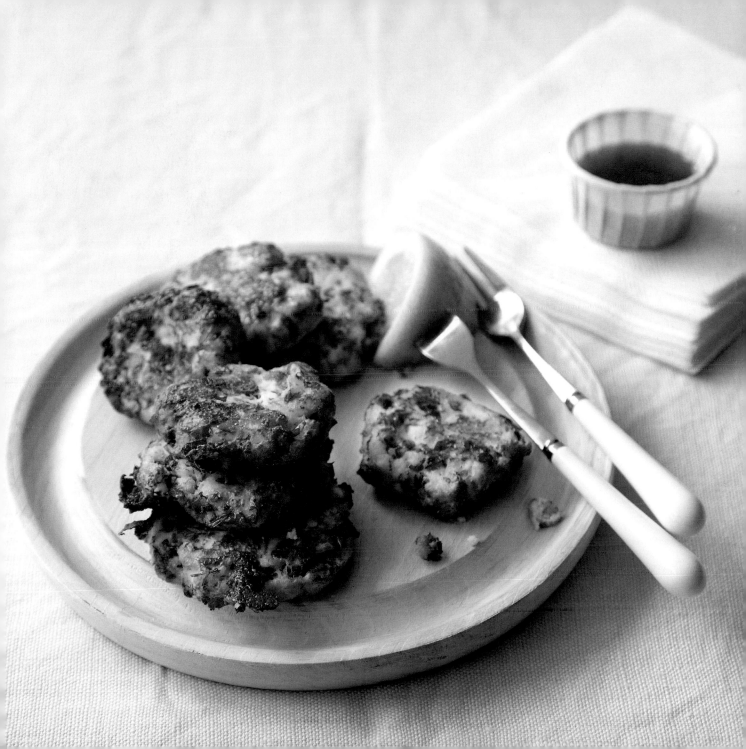

Pumpkin and Egg Curry

This delicious southern Indian-style curry can be eaten on its own as a stew or ladled over a thick bed of lightly buttered leaf spinach (cooked from fresh or frozen). Ordinary "jack-o-lantern"-type pumpkins have the lightest carb ratio; dense orange-fleshed squashes, such as butternut and kabocha, will work beautifully, although they do have a slightly higher carbohydrate count.

For the spice paste
3 garlic cloves
2.5 cm/1 inch piece of fresh
    root ginger, grated
1 tsp coriander seeds
1 tsp cumin seeds
½ tsp ground turmeric
1 tsp chilli flakes
½ tsp sea salt

2 tbsp sunflower oil
200 g/7 oz pumpkin,
    peeled, de-seeded and
    cut into chunks
200 g/7 oz courgettes,
    cut into chunks
125 g/4 oz celery, sliced
400 g/14 oz can coconut milk
200 g/7 oz canned chopped
    tomatoes
Sea salt and freshly ground
    black pepper
4 organic eggs
Chopped coriander, to garnish
    (optional)

Serves 4

First, make the spice paste. Place all ingredients in a blender or spice grinder. Add enough water to allow the blades to run smoothly and process until a smooth, pourable paste results.

Heat a wok or large pan over a medium heat. Add the oil and, when it's hot, add the pumpkin, courgettes and celery, and stir-fry for about 2 minutes, until starting to soften. Pour in the spice paste and stir briskly for 1–2 minutes, until fragrant and evenly distributed. Add the coconut milk and tomatoes, and season well with salt and pepper. Bring·to the boil, then lower the heat to a simmer. Cook, stirring frequently, for about 30 minutes, until the pumpkin has softened so much that it begins to melt into the thick curry sauce.

Meanwhile, cook the eggs. Place them in a small pan and cover with cold water. Bring to the boil and cook for 7 minutes, then drain and cool under cold running water. Crack and remove the shell and slice in half.

When the curry is cooked, stir well, then lay the egg halves on the surface of the curry. Simmer for 2 minutes, without stirring, until the eggs are warmed through. Sprinkle coriander leaves over the curry and serve.

Per serving
Carbs: 8 g protein: 12 g calories: 344 fibre: 1.5 g fat: 30 g (saturated fat: 3 g)

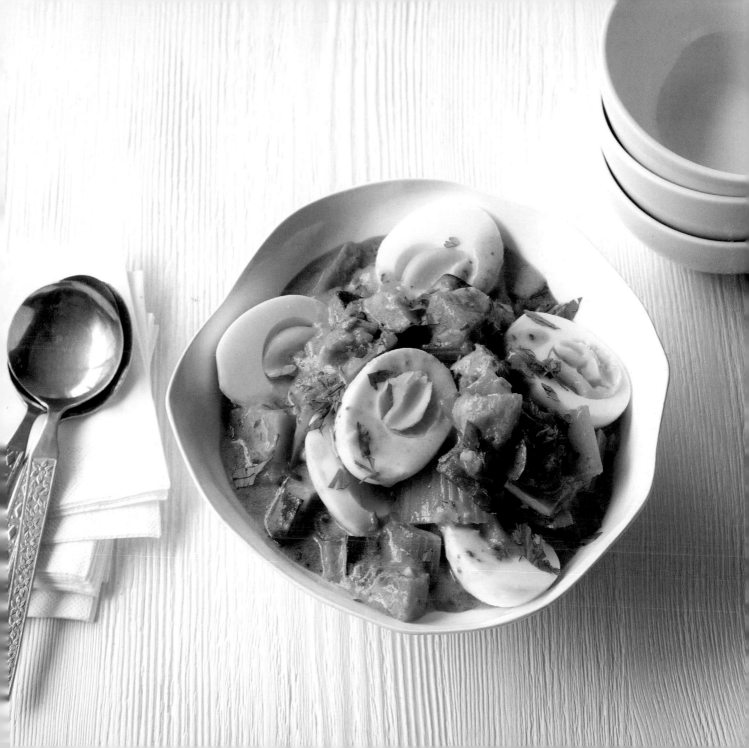

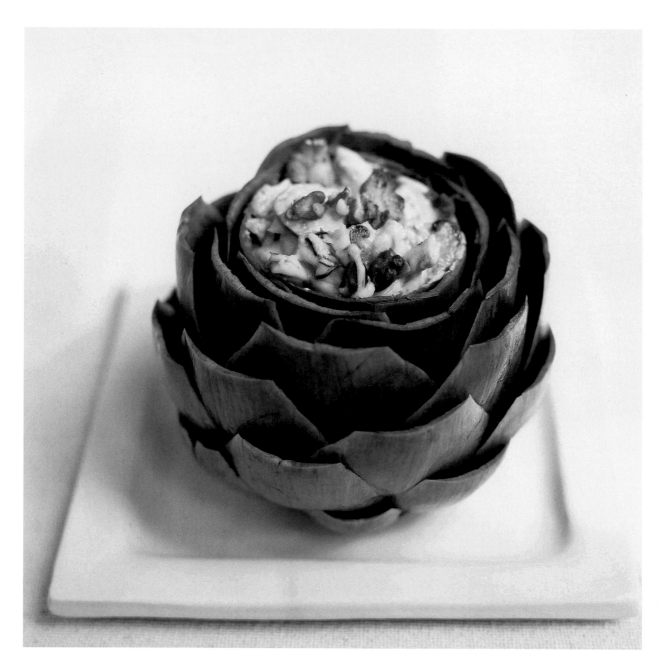

Artichokes Stuffed with Creamy Wild Mushrooms

You might call this "gilding the lily" – it's hard to improve on the perfect globe artichoke, boiled whole and served with melted butter or mayonnaise. This recipe does elevate it, however, not only to red-carpet status, but renders it a complete meal with minimum effort. Enjoy.

2 tbsp white wine vinegar

2 tbsp olive oil

15 g/½ oz/1 tbsp butter

4 large fresh globe artichokes

300 g/11 oz mixed wild mushrooms (especially morels, chanterelles and ceps), chopped into small chunks

2 tsp fresh thyme or lemon thyme leaves

5 tbsp dry vermouth

150 g/5 oz mascarpone cheese

50 g/2 oz walnuts, crushed

A handful of flat-leaf parsley leaves, chopped

Salt and freshly ground black pepper

Serves 4

Bring a large pan of water to the boil. Add the vinegar, olive oil and plenty of salt to the water.

Meanwhile, prepare the artichokes. Cut off the stems flush with the base, and slice about one-third off the top. Pull out what you can from the middle and use a spoon to scoop out all of the hairy choke. Place in the boiling water and cook for 30–40 minutes, until tender. They are done when a leaf pulled from near the centre comes away without resistance. Drain, and use tongs to turn upside down in the colander until dry. Preheat the oven to 220°C/425°F/Gas Mark 7.

To make the stuffing, melt the butter in a wide frying pan over a medium heat and add the mushrooms and thyme with a sprinkling of salt and pepper. When they have absorbed the butter and begin to soften, pour in the vermouth and cook, stirring, until it has almost all evaporated. Finally, stir in the mascarpone. Stir until the mushrooms are evenly coated.

Place the artichokes, bottom down, on a lined baking tray. Spoon the mixture into the middle of the drained artichokes. Sprinkle with crushed walnuts and bake for 10–15 minutes, until heated through and golden on top. Garnish with chopped parsley before serving. When eating, use the leaves of the artichoke to scoop out the creamy filling.

Per serving
Carbs: 3.5 g protein: 6.5 g calories: 324 fibre: 1 g fat: 30 g (saturated fat: 14 g)

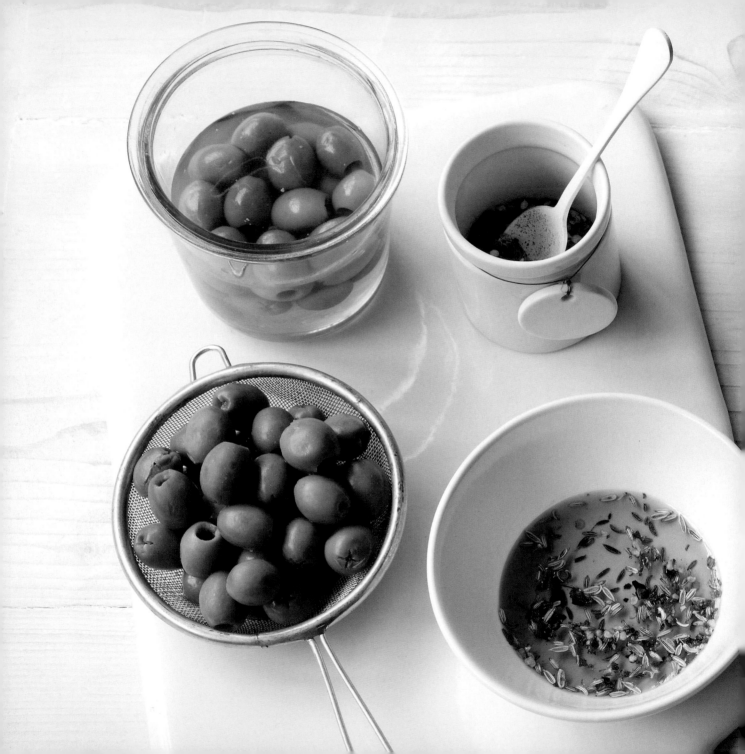

05:
NIBBLES
SNACKS
AND QUICK FIXES

It used to be so easy to reach for a sandwich or a bag of chips –
low-carb life is different. A mouthful of impact-flavoured protein
or tasty, vitamin-packed veggies are the solution, and it's still easy.

Chilli-Crust Brazil Nuts

Roasting brings out the best flavour in nuts, and these have an added dimension with the flavourful chilli crust. When roasting nuts, it's essential to use a timer, as the short cooking time means they so easily get forgotten.

1 tbsp olive oil
2 tsp dark soy sauce
1 tsp lemon juice
1 tsp sweetener
1 tsp paprika
½ tsp crushed chilli flakes
1 tsp sesame seeds
150 g/5 oz Brazil nuts

Serves 8

Preheat the oven to 190°C/375°F/Gas Mark 5. Whisk together all the ingredients except the Brazil nuts. Stir in the nuts and coat evenly. Spread them out in a single layer on a baking sheet and roast, stirring every 2 minutes, until golden, about 10 minutes in total.

Cool completely, then transfer to a bowl and serve. Store in an airtight container.

Per serving
Carbs: 0.6 g protein: 2.6 g calories: 141 fibre: 0.8 g fat: 14 g (saturated fat: 3.2 g)

Olive Raisins

Virtually carbohydrate-free, olives are a great snack. This roasting technique gives them pleasingly chewy texture. Feel free to experiment with different spices – fennel seeds give a fragrant crunch.

200 g/7 oz large stoned green olives
½ tsp fennel seeds
½ tsp chilli flakes
2 tbsp olive oil

Serves 4

Preheat the oven to 200°C/400°F/Gas Mark 6. Place the olives in a small ovenproof dish and stir in the remaining ingredients to coat evenly. Roast for 25–30 minutes, until shrunken and wrinkly. Leave to cool before serving.

Per serving
Carbs: 0 g protein: 0.5 g calories: 100 fibre: 1.5 g fat: 11 g (saturated fat: 1.5 g)

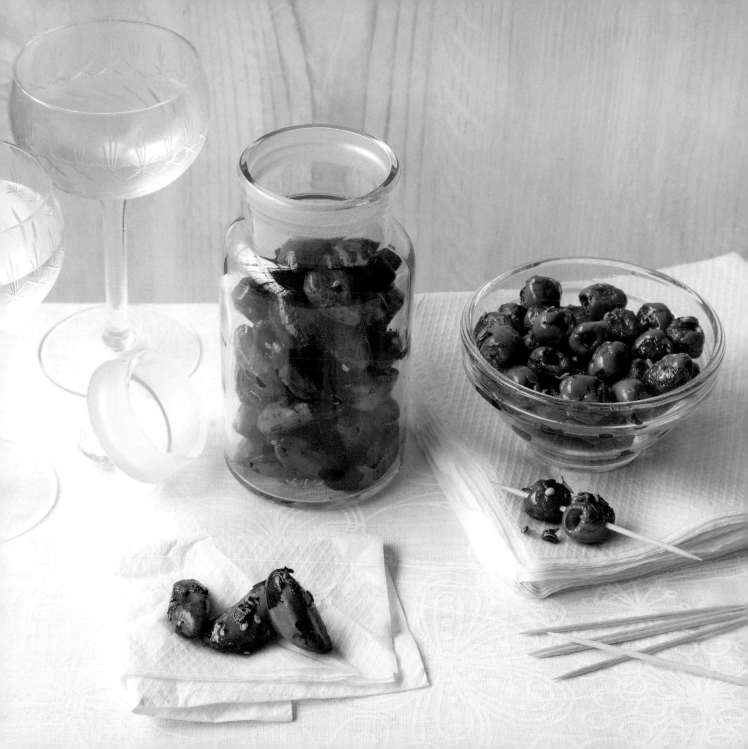

Edam Crisps

This method can be applied to some other hard cheeses, including Gouda, but in my experience, Edam gets the best results every time. A reliable non-stick pan is the only tool for the job. Pre-sliced cheese is recommended, as it may be more thinly sliced than you can manage yourself. Check the label if you are concerned about non-vegetarian rennet in the Edam.

100 g/3½ oz Edam cheese,
    sliced into 8 very thin pieces

Makes 8

Lay the cheese slices in a non-stick pan, leaving a space of at least 1 cm/½ inch between them. You may have to cook in batches if your pan is too small. Place the pan over the lowest possible heat.

The cheese will bubble and pop, oil will ooze out, and eventually the cheese will start to turn crisp underneath. Cook until the underside is looking dry and very slightly golden. This may take up to 15 minutes. Turn the cheese over carefully and cook the other side for about 5 minutes until crisp. Drain the cheese crisps on kitchen paper. Serve warm or cold.

Per serving
Carbs: 0 g protein: 3 g calories: 43 fibre: 0 g fat: 3 g (saturated fat: 2 g)

Parmesan Wafers

These feather-light savoury wafers are best enjoyed straight out of the oven or soon afterwards. They soften slightly as they cool, but can be re-crisped in the oven later (4–5 minutes at 180°C/350°F/Gas Mark 4). Seek out a vegetarian Parmesan substitute if you are concerned about animal rennet.

2 organic egg whites
Pinch of cream of tartar
3 tbsp finely grated Parmesan cheese

Makes 8

Preheat the oven to 150°C/300°F/Gas Mark 2. Beat the egg whites with the cream of tartar in a grease-free bowl until stiff but not dry. Gently fold in the Parmesan, keeping the mixture light and airy, until evenly incorporated. Spoon on to a parchment-lined baking sheet to make 8 wafers and bake for about 15 minutes, until golden and crisp.

Per serving
Carbs: 0 g protein: 1.5 g calories: 13 fibre: 0 g fat: 0.7 g (saturated fat: 0.5 g)

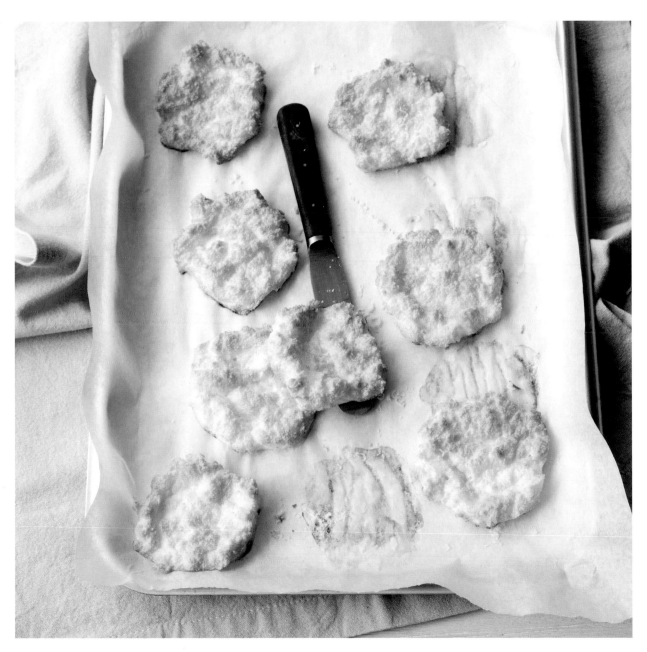

Mexican Cucumbers

I was first introduced to these in Mexico, where they are served as bar snacks – it's a surprisingly good combination. The mild chilli powder I use is a commonly sold mixture with added garlic powder and oregano. A pre-made "taco seasoning" also works well.

1 medium cucumber,
  about 300 g/11 oz
2 limes
2 tsp mild chilli powder mix
  or taco seasoning mix
Sea salt

Serves 8

Trim the ends of the cucumber, then cut it across into four pieces of equal length. Cut each piece lengthways into eight wedges. Arrange the wedges skin-side down in a dish and squeeze the juice from the limes over them. Sprinkle with an even coat of mild chilli powder and season with salt.

Per serving
Carbs: 0.5 g protein: 0.3 g calories: 4 fibre: 0.3 g fat: 0 g (saturated fat: 0 g)

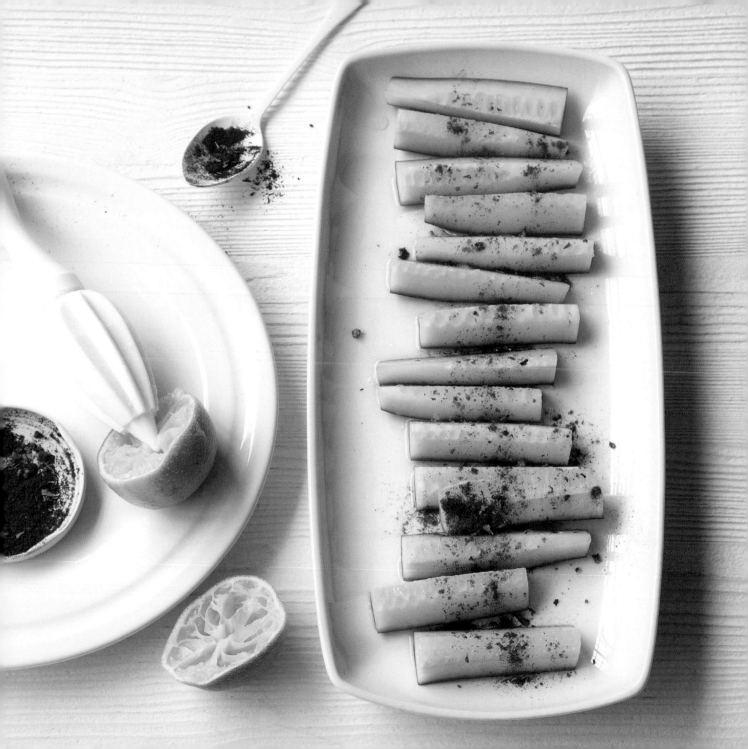

Spicy Tofu Biltong

Deeply flavoured and toothsome, these do a surprisingly good job of imitating beef jerky or biltong.

200 g smoked or plain tofu
    (flavoured or pre-marinated
    can also be used)
2 tbsp dark soy sauce
2 tbsp dry sherry
1 tsp rice vinegar
Pinch of cayenne pepper
1 tbsp sunflower oil

Makes 14

Preheat the oven to 120°C/250°F/Gas Mark ½. Pat the tofu dry with kitchen paper, then slice very thinly into about 14 strips, about 2.5 cm/1 inch wide, 7.5 cm/3 inches long and roughly 3 mm/⅛ inch thick.

Line a baking sheet with non-stick baking parchment. Thoroughly whisk all the remaining ingredients together in a shallow dish. Dip each piece of tofu in the mixture, then lay on the baking sheet. Spoon any remaining mixture carefully over the tofu strips.

Place in the oven and cook for about 60–80 minutes, until the tofu is crisp around the edges, but still pliable. Leave to cool. The strips can be stored in an airtight container in the refrigerator for up to 3 days.

Per serving
Carbs: 0.3 g protein: 1 g calories: 21 fibre: 0 g fat: 1.5 g (saturated fat: 0.2 g)

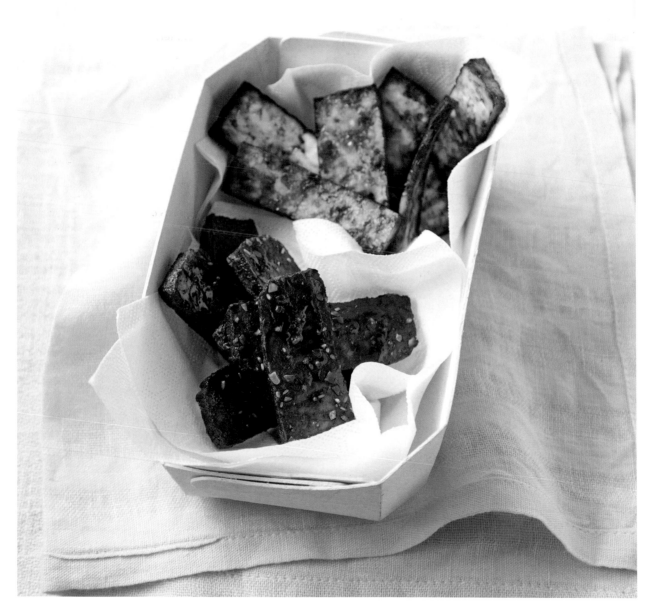

Sesame and
Black Pepper Crispbreads

When you really miss that cracker-crunch, these are a godsend. Cooking this batter in a microwave seems to be the only way to get a super-crisp result. They are a great companion to the soups in this book.

2 tbsp sesame seeds

Olive oil, for brushing

50 g/2 oz soy flour

1 organic egg

½ tsp salt

120 ml/4 fl oz warm water

1 tsp freshly ground black pepper

Makes 8

First toast the sesame seeds. Heat a dry frying pan over a medium heat. Add the sesame seeds and toast, stirring frequently, until golden and popping. Remove from the pan and set aside.

Line a microwave-safe plate with non-stick baking parchment. Brush it generously with olive oil. Beat together the flour, egg, salt, water and pepper until smooth. Pour a thin layer of batter on to the plate, about 6 cm/2½ inches in diameter. Sprinkle with sesame seeds. Microwave on high for 1½–3 minutes, until dry and crisp. Cooking time will depend on the microwave. Cool on a wire rack. Repeat with the remaining batter. Store in an airtight container.

Per serving
Carbs: 1.5 g protein: 4 g calories: 65 fibre: 1 g fat: 5 g (saturated fat: 0.8 g)

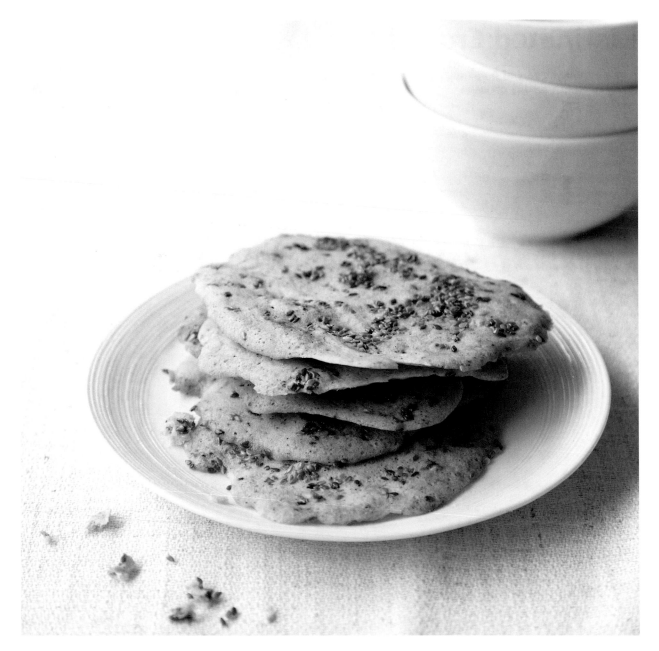

Marinated Crudité Salad

Here's a fantastic way of preparing raw vegetables which will keep in the refrigerator for a few days, ready to munch on any occasion.

½ red pepper, cored
½ yellow pepper, cored
100 g/3½ oz sugar snap peas
100 g/3½ oz fine green beans,
    trimmed
50 g/2 oz courgette
50 g/2 oz celery
100 g/3½ oz fennel
1 tbsp sea salt
1 tbsp lemon juice
1 tbsp extra-virgin olive oil

Serves 4

If the vegetable lends itself to being cut into strips, do so; others can be cut into similar size pieces (for example, beans and fennel).

Place them all in a bowl and sprinkle with the salt. Toss with your hands to coat evenly. Transfer to a colander and place over a bowl which will fit in the fridge. Cover with clingfilm and refrigerate, stirring occasionally, for 3–4 hours.

Shake the veg in the colander to drain thoroughly (do not rinse). Place the veg in a clean bowl, add lemon juice and olive oil, and stir. Store covered in the fridge, ideally in a plastic container with a tight-fitting lid so you can shake occasionally, bringing the flavourful juices back up to dress the veg.

Per serving
Carbs: 5 g protein: 2 g calories: 57 fibre: 2.5 g fat: 3 g (saturated fat: 0.5 g)

Celery with Pesto

Here's an easy solution when you're in the mood to raid the refrigerator. You can use ready-made pesto or make your own (see p.165).

2 celery sticks, trimmed

2 tbsp cream cheese

1–2 tsp pesto

Freshly ground black pepper

Serves 2

Use a butter knife to spread the cream cheese inside the curve of the celery. Drizzle pesto down the middle. Grind over some pepper, then eat whole or slice diagonally into bite-size pieces.

Per serving
Carbs: 0.4 g protein: 0.6 g calories: 70 fibre: 0.3 g fat: 7 g (saturated fat: 4 g)

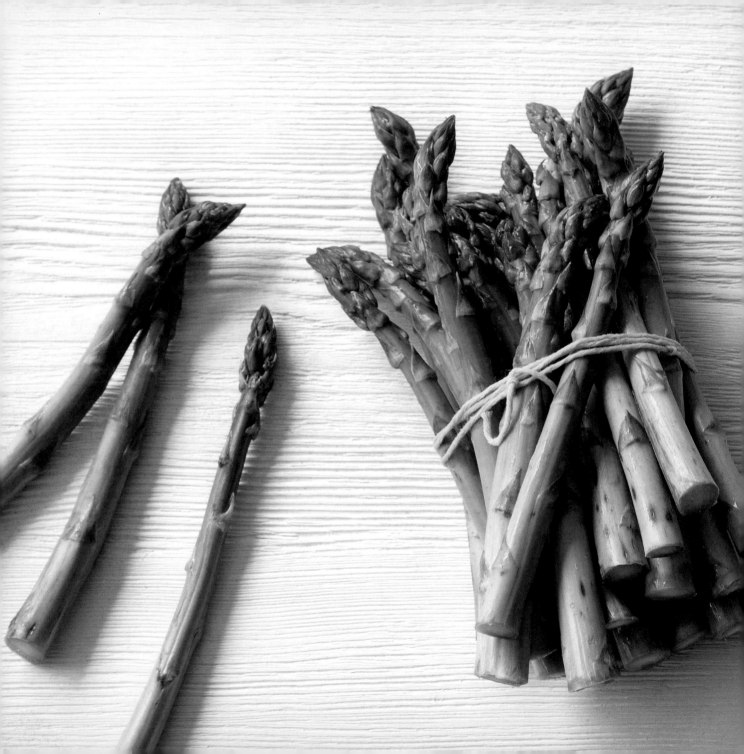

06:
PARTY FOOD

Canapés and finger food should be easy to make, easy to eat, beautiful, luxurious, and moreish. It's all possible with this chapter. Enjoy with champagne or vodka martinis.

Aubergine
and Smoked Cheese Involtini

Involtini are simply "little rolls" in Italian. In this case, chargrilled aubergine slices encase little rod-shaped pieces of melting smoked cheese, which ideally should be a smoked mozzarella, but as it's rather a privilege to come across the real thing, any smoked cheese will do. Pictured here with Green Bean and Roasted Red Pepper Parcels (see p.116).

2 aubergines,
    about 600 g/1 lb 5oz,
    stem removed and sliced
    lengthways as thinly as possible
4 tbsp olive oil
25 large fresh basil leaves
100 g/3½ oz smoked mozzarella,
    smoked Cheddar or other smoked
    cheese, cut in 25 pieces, measuring
    about 20 x 5 mm/¾ x ¼ inches
Sea salt and freshly ground
    black pepper

Makes 25

Heat a chargrill pan for about 10 minutes, until very hot. Brush the aubergine slices lightly on both sides with olive oil. Cook on the chargrill pan until soft and striped with black on both sides. Season each slice with salt and pepper and leave to cool.

Place a basil leaf at one end of an aubergine slice and a piece of cheese on top of the basil. Roll the slice up around the cheese and basil. Place, seam-side down, on a baking sheet. Repeat with the remaining ingredients.

Preheat the oven to 200°/400°F/Gas Mark 6. Just before serving, put the involtini in the oven for no longer than 5 minutes just to warm through – it's best to set a timer or they might overcook if forgotten. Serve warm and melting.

Per serving
Carbs: 0.5 g protein: 1 g calories: 30 fibre: 0.5 g fat: 3 g (saturated fat: 1 g)

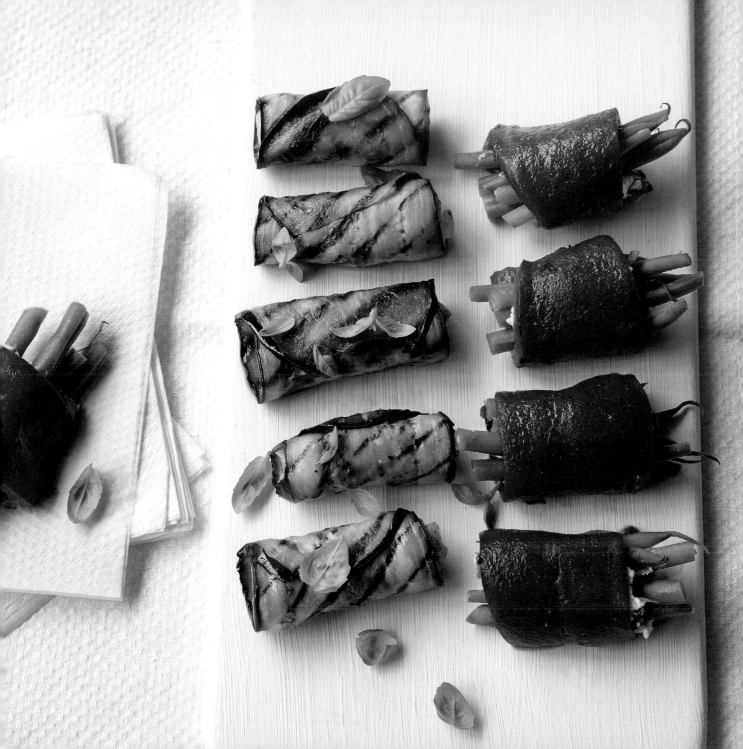

Green Bean
and Roasted Pepper Parcels

Simplicity itself, beautiful to behold, and even more gorgeous to eat. Don't save these just for a party – you should spoil yourself and your family with them, too, as a neat little appetiser or accompaniment. If you're really pushed for time, use grilled peppers from a jar, can, or deli – although fresh always tastes best. Pictured on p.115.

2 red peppers
100 g/3½ oz fine green beans, trimmed
50 g/2 oz cream cheese
8 fresh basil leaves, shredded
Sea salt and freshly ground black pepper

Makes 8

Preheat the grill to its highest setting. Cut the peppers in half from stem to base and remove the cores and stems. Place, cut-side down, on a baking sheet lined with non-stick parchment. Grill the peppers until blackened and blistered all over. Remove to a plastic bag and seal. Leave to cool.

Meanwhile, bring a small pan of water to the boil and add salt. Cook the green beans for 2–3 minutes, until just tender but still bright green. Drain and cool under cold running water. Pat dry.

Peel the skins carefully off the peppers, taking care not to tear the flesh. Cut each half in half again from stem end to base. Lay on a board, peeled-side down. Place about a rounded teaspoonful of cream cheese on the surface of each piece, then sprinkle basil over the cheese. Grind a little salt and pepper over them. Lay a bundle of 4–5 green beans across the top and wrap the pepper around the beans. Place seam-side down on a plate and chill in the refrigerator until ready to serve.

Per serving
Carbs: 3 g protein: 1 g calories: 48 fibre: 1 g fat: 4 g (saturated fat: 2 g)

Tricolore Skewers

The three colours of the Italian flag, in one bite, on a skewer. Use buffalo milk mozzarella for the creamiest flavour; failing that, cow's milk, but always from a snow-white ball, not the "pizza cheese" type.

1 buffalo mozzarella,
　　torn into 24 bite-size shreds
24 semi-dried, sunblush or
　　sun-dried tomatoes in oil
24 large fresh basil leaves

Makes 24

Pair up a piece of mozzarella and a tomato. Wrap a basil leaf around them and secure with a medium bamboo skewer. Serve immediately.

Per serving
Carbs: 0.1 g protein: 1.5 g calories: 29 fibre: 0 g fat: 2.5 g (saturated fat: 1 g)

Cucumber
with Pink Pickled Ginger

Pink pickled ginger is an essential accompaniment for sushi and can be found in Asian groceries and health-food shops. Look out for the shredded psychedelic fuchsia type (you can't miss it!), for maximum visual impact, or use the traditional light pink type. Pictured on p.119.

1 quantity Satay Sauce (see p.169)
Half a cucumber
　　(about 13 cm/ 5 inches,
　　200 g/7 oz)
50 g/4 tbsp pink pickled ginger
1 spring onion,
　　finely sliced diagonally

Makes 20

Cool the Satay Sauce, then chill until thick.

Peel the cucumber and cut into 20 slices, 5 mm/¼ inch thick. (If desired, you can make neat shapes with a small cookie cutter.)

Spoon a small dollop of Satay Sauce on each piece, then top with a pinch of pickled ginger. Garnish with a slice of spring onion.

Per serving
Carbs: 0.6 g protein: 0.6 g calories: 16 fibre: 0.2 g fat: 1 g (saturated fat: 0.3 g)

Cucumber and Tofu Satay

On a day-to-day basis, I wouldn't normally fuss around threading bits on to skewers for supper, which is why this recipe lands in the Party Food chapter. However, I think you'll find these are easy and tasty enough to enjoy without a special occasion. Freezing the tofu gives it a remarkable fibrous texture which resembles chicken – try the technique below in other tofu dishes. Or simply use fresh firm tofu. Pictured here with Cucumber with Pink Pickled Ginger (see p.117)

100 g/3½ oz firm tofu

100 g/3½ oz cucumber

1 quantity Satay Sauce
(see p.169)

1 quantity Sweet Chilli Sauce
(see p.166) (optional)

Makes 12

Freeze the tofu until completely solid, then thaw completely before using. Drain thoroughly and wrap in kitchen paper. Place on a plate and weigh down with a heavy object, such as a pan of water – this will compress the tofu slightly and squeeze out excess moisture. Leave for about 30 minutes, then cut into small cubes, about 1 cm/½ inch wide.

Cut the cucumber into strips the same width and remove the seeds. Cut into pieces the same size as the tofu. Thread alternating pieces of tofu and cucumber on to 12 medium-length bamboo skewers, using three of each per skewer. Lay the skewers side by side on a plate. Spoon Satay Sauce generously over them and serve, adding Sweet Chilli Sauce if desired.

Per serving
Carbs: 1 g protein: 2 g calories: 32 fibre: 0.5 g fat: 2.5 g (saturated fat: 0.5 g)

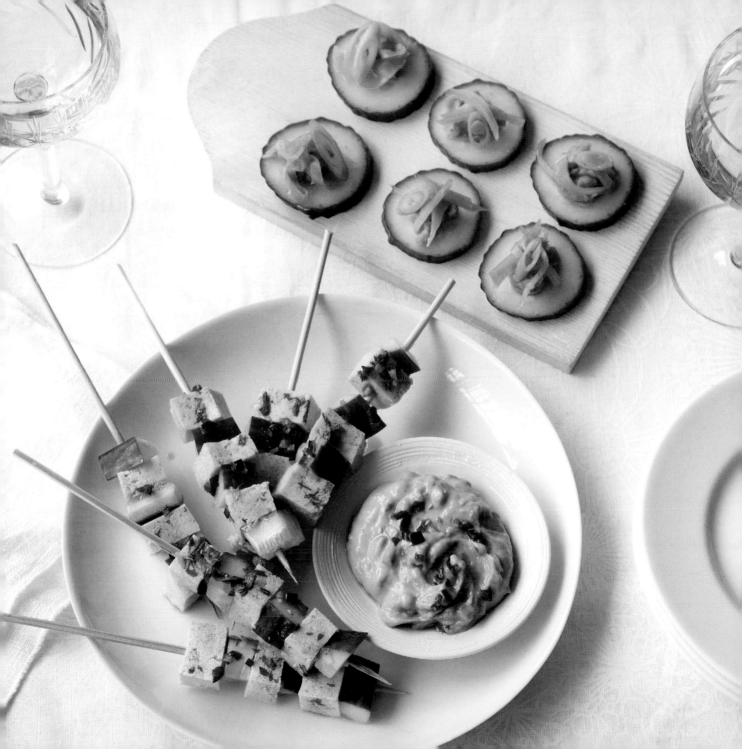

Saffron Aïoli
with Quail's Eggs and Asparagus

Quail's eggs are wonderfully elegant, but undeniably awkward to peel. They are so beautiful in the shell, I always leave it on and let the guests do the work.

24 quail's eggs

3 bunches asparagus,
	woody ends snapped off

5 garlic cloves (or to taste), central
	sprouts removed, if any

3 organic egg yolks

½ tsp saffron threads,
	soaked in 1 tbsp hot water

Salt

250 ml/8 fl oz light olive oil

2 tbsp lemon juice

Serves 8

Place the quail's eggs in a pan and cover with cold water. Bring to the boil and cook for 3 minutes. Drain and cool under cold running water until completely cold.

Steam the asparagus until barely tender, or cooked to your liking. Cool.

Put the garlic in a food processor and process until finely chopped. Add the egg yolks, soaked saffron and soaking water, and a little salt in a food processor and process to combine. With the motor running, add the oil, one drop at a time. Gradually increase the pace and pour in the remaining oil in a very thin, steady stream until a thick mayonnaise is achieved. If the aïoli curdles, add another egg yolk.

Beat in the lemon juice. Scoop into a bowl and serve on a platter with quail's eggs and asparagus.

Per serving
Carbs: 1.5 g protein: 13 g calories: 365 fibre: 1.3 g fat: 34 g (saturated fat: 6 g)

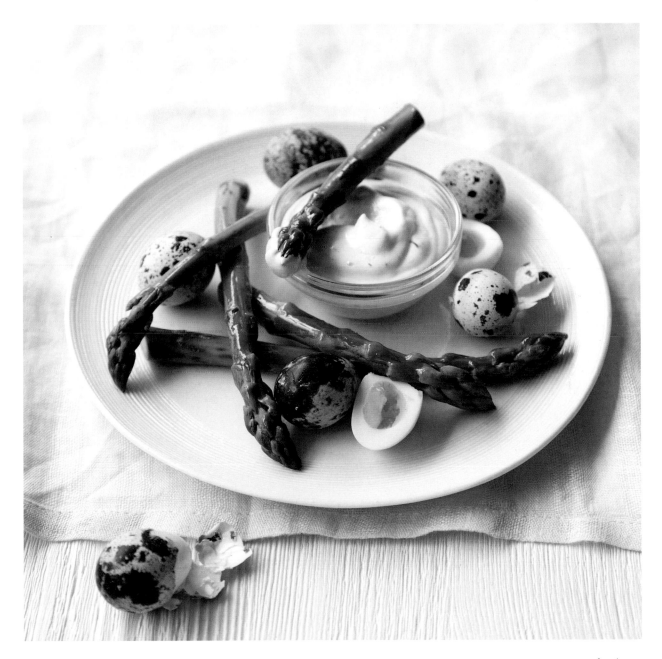

Chilli Citrus Labneh Platter

"Labneh" is a Middle Eastern soft fresh cheese made by transforming yogurt overnight in your refrigerator. It couldn't be simpler and you can flavour it with whatever you like – fresh or dried herbs, or whole toasted spices such as cumin. This red chilli and citrus version is particularly pretty and the flavour just dances on the tongue. Be sure you remove only the outer zest of the orange and lemon and none of the bitter white pith.

500 ml/18 fl oz Greek yogurt
    or other full-fat yogurt
2 hot red chillies, chopped
grated zest of 1 orange
grated zest of 1 lemon
extra-virgin olive oil,
    for drizzling
Salt

To serve
About 500 g/ 1¼ lb raw vegetables,
    such as celery sticks, pepper strips,
    cucumber batons, sugar snap peas

Serves 8

Line a small, fine strainer with a piece of muslin, cheesecloth, or a new kitchen cloth. The shape of your strainer will determine the shape of the *labneh* – a conical shape is attractive. Set the strainer over a deep bowl so there is plenty of space for the whey to drain away, and make sure there is room for it in your refrigerator.

Mix the yogurt thoroughly with the chillies, citrus zests and a generous pinch of salt for maximum flavour. Scoop the mixture into the strainer and smooth down. Cover with clingfilm and place in the refrigerator for 24–36 hours. Turn out on to a plate and drizzle with olive oil. Arrange the vegetables around the *labneh* and serve, with a butter knife for spreading.

Per serving
Carbs: 3 g protein: 3 g calories: 58 fibre: 0 g fat: 4 g (saturated fat: 2.5 g)

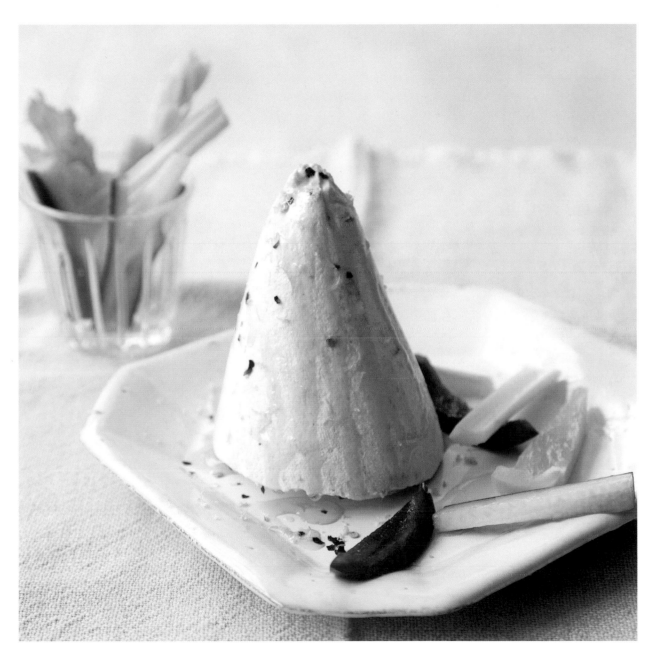

Hot Artichoke Sin

I call this "Sin" as a reminder that it is pure indulgence; that's also why it resides in the Party Food chapter. It is not particularly elegant-looking, but the taste never fails to please.

**400 g/14 oz can artichoke hearts,
  drained and chopped**
120 ml/4 fl oz mayonnaise
**50 g/2 oz freshly grated
  Parmesan cheese**
**2 large green chillies,
  de-seeded and chopped**
1 organic egg

Serves 8

Preheat the oven to 220°C/425°F/Gas Mark 7. Mix together the artichoke hearts, mayonnaise, cheese and chillies in a bowl. Beat in the egg. Spread into a wide ovenproof dish in a layer no more than 2 cm/¾ inch deep.

Bake the mixture for about 30 minutes, until bubbling and very dark golden on top and bottom. Remove from the oven and leave to cool.

To serve, slide on to a board and cut into bite-size squares with a knife or pizza-cutter.

Per serving
Carbs: 5 g protein: 5 g calories: 176 fibre: 2 g fat: 15 g (saturated fat: 3.5 g)

Smoked Aubergine Purée

This dip is also known as *Baba Ganoush*. Cooking the aubergine directly over a naked flame gives it a mystical smoky flavour, while softening it to a pulp. If you don't cook on gas, see instructions on how to oven-cook, below.

2 medium aubergines

1 garlic clove

2 tbsp lemon juice

2 tbsp extra-virgin olive oil

3 tbsp Greek yogurt

Coarse salt and freshly ground
    black pepper

To serve

About 500 g/1¼ lb raw vegetables,
    such as celery sticks, pepper strips,
    cucumber batons, Little Gem
    lettuce leaves, chicory leaves

Serves 8

Push a fork into the stem of an aubergine and hold directly in a high gas flame. Turn occasionally until completely soft and collapsed; the skin should be blackened to the point of ash in places, and steam should be escaping through the fork holes. Repeat with the second aubergine. Alternatively, preheat the oven to its highest setting. Prick the aubergines a few times, place on a baking sheet and roast until completely soft.

Remove to a plate and leave to cool. Peel off the charred skins. Don't worry if a few little charred flecks remain as they will add to the flavour. Place the flesh in a bowl.

Crush the garlic clove with a little coarse salt in a mortar with a pestle for the best flavour. Alternatively, use a garlic crusher. Using a fork, break up the aubergines, then mash together with the crushed garlic and remaining ingredients, until fairly smooth. Season to taste.

Per serving

Carbs: 2 g protein: 1 g calories: 41 fibre: 1.5 g fat: 3.5 g (saturated fat: 0.7 g)

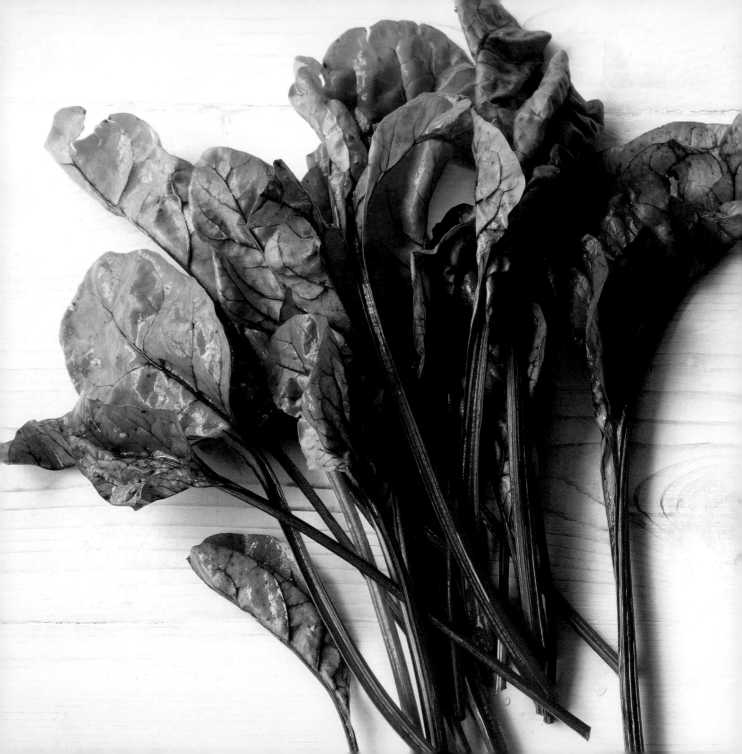

07:
ON THE SIDE

The best vegetarian food is a balanced composition of flavours and textures on the plate. None of these recipes need play second fiddle, but become part of a richly varied menu when paired up with other dishes.

Avocado and Lemon Salad

Small pieces of whole lemon and a ginger-spiked dressing complement the creamy, rich avocado. Serve this with Red Pepper and Goat's Cheese Timbales (see p.45).

1 lemon

2 ripe avocados

Sea salt, to taste

1 tsp finely grated fresh root ginger

4 tbsp extra-virgin olive oil

4 handfuls young spinach leaves,
   about 100 g/3½ oz

Serves 4

Halve the lemon. Squeeze and strain the juice from one half into a small jug for the dressing. Cut the other in half again and then slice as thinly as possible.

Peel, halve and stone the avocados. Cut them into quarters, then slice.

Mix the salt and ginger into the lemon juice, then gradually whisk in the olive oil.

Arrange the spinach leaves on a platter or individual plates. Place the avocado and lemon slices on top. Drizzle the dressing over them and serve immediately.

Per serving
Carbs: 2 g protein: 2.5 g calories: 247 fibre: 3 g fat: 25 g (saturated fat: 4 g)

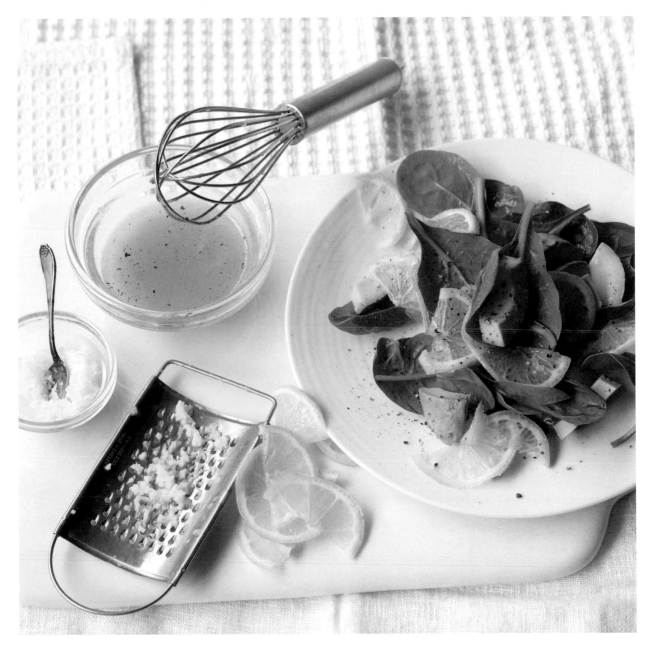

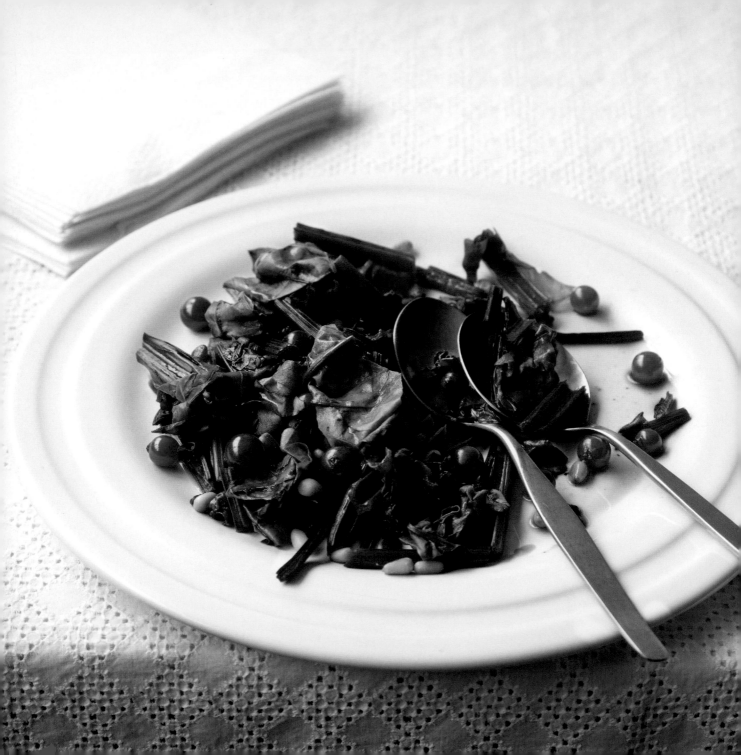

Ruby Chard
with Pine Nuts and Redcurrants

Tart, blushing redcurrants are sublime with the earthy chard; a handful of cranberries could be substituted off-season – add them to the pan with the pine nuts. Serve this with Aubergine Rarebit (see p.50) or Creamy Celeriac Gratin (see p.76).

500 g/1 lb ruby chard with stalks,
    or beetroot greens or Swiss chard
2 tbsp olive oil
25 g/1 oz pine nuts
50 g/2 oz redcurrants
Salt and freshly ground black pepper

Serves 2–4

Wash and dry the chard or greens, strip the leaves and chop coarsely. Chop the stalks into 2 cm/¾ inch wide pieces.

Heat the oil in a pan and add the pine nuts. Cook, stirring, until the nuts are golden. Add the chard stalks, season with salt and pepper, and stir. Cover the pan and cook, stirring occasionally, for about 3 minutes, until softened. Add chopped leaves, cover and cook until just wilted.

Transfer the mixture to a platter using a slotted spoon and sprinkle with the redcurrants.

Per serving
Carbs: 4 g protein: 3 g calories: 119 fibre: 0.5 g fat: 10 g (saturated fat: 1 g)

Braised Fennel and Peppers

This bold and rustic Mediterranean side dish is the ideal foil for Rocket and Ricotta Cheesecake (see p.72), Roasted Aubergines with Dill Sauce (see p.133), or an omelette.

3 tbsp olive oil

2 fennel bulbs, trimmed and sliced

1 red pepper, cored and sliced

1 yellow pepper, cored and sliced

3–4 fresh thyme sprigs

1 tsp coriander seeds

1 tsp chilli flakes

10 green queen olives

2 garlic cloves, crushed

120 ml/4 fl oz red wine

Salt and freshly ground black pepper

Serves 4

Heat the oil in a wide frying pan over a medium heat and add the fennel, peppers and thyme. Cook, stirring frequently, until the vegetables are beginning to soften and brown.

Add the coriander seeds, chilli flakes and olives, season with salt and pepper, and cook for a further 5 minutes. Add the garlic and cook very briefly until fragrant, then add the wine. Simmer until the liquid has evaporated.

Per serving
Carbs: 6 g protein: 1 g calories: 136 fibre: 3 g fat: 10 g (saturated fat: 1.5 g)

Roasted Aubergines with Dill Sauce

Here, the hot aubergines are doused in a cool, creamy sauce to create a warm salad – very nice in its own right, with crunchy lettuce leaves. Also try it with Halloumi-Stuffed Peppers (see p.48) or Braised Fennel and Peppers (see p.132).

2 large aubergines

Olive oil, for brushing

250 ml/8 fl oz Greek yogurt

3 tbsp chopped fresh dill,
    or 2 tbsp freeze-dried dill

Grated rind of 1 lemon

Juice of ½ lemon

1 small garlic clove, crushed

Salt and freshly ground black pepper

Serves 4

Preheat the oven to 220°C/425°F/Gas Mark 7. Chop the stems off the aubergines and cut into six long wedges from top to bottom. Score the flesh diagonally without piercing the skin. Brush generously with olive oil and place, flesh side down, in a roasting tin. Season with salt and pepper. Roast for about 30 minutes, until soft and tinged with gold.

Meanwhile, make the sauce. Combine all the remaining ingredients thoroughly. Spoon the sauce over the hot aubergines and serve.

Per serving
Carbs: 4 g protein: 4 g calories: 115 fibre: 1 g fat: 9 g (saturated fat: 5 g)

Turnip Dauphinoise

I scanned dozens of French cookbooks searching for the ultimate Potato Dauphinoise recipe, but in the end I took a cue from stylish London cook Alastair Hendy, who makes a warm cream infusion and adds chives to his. Believe me, low-carb turnips plug into this classic dish like they were always meant to be there. To make life easy, use a food processor with a slicing blade for the turnips if you can. Celeriac can be substituted for turnips, without gaining any carbs.

15 g/½ oz/1 tbsp butter,
    for greasing
1 kg/2¼ lb turnips, trimmed weight,
    peeled and thinly sliced
Sea salt and freshly ground
    black pepper
1 large bunch of chives, chopped
1 garlic clove, halved
250 ml/8 fl oz double cream
250 ml/8 fl oz sour cream
100 ml/3½ fl oz water

Serves 6

Preheat the oven to 160°C/325°F/Gas Mark 3. Butter a medium-sized gratin dish.

Make layers of turnip slices, sprinkling with salt, pepper and chives as you go.

Place the garlic, cream, sour cream and water in a small pan. Gradually bring to just before boiling point, stirring constantly, then remove from the heat. Pour the mixture over the turnips and discard the garlic.

Bake for 1¼–1½ hours, until the turnips are fork-tender throughout.

Per serving
Carbs: 10 g protein: 3 g calories: 349 fibre: 4 g fat: 33 g (saturated fat: 20 g)

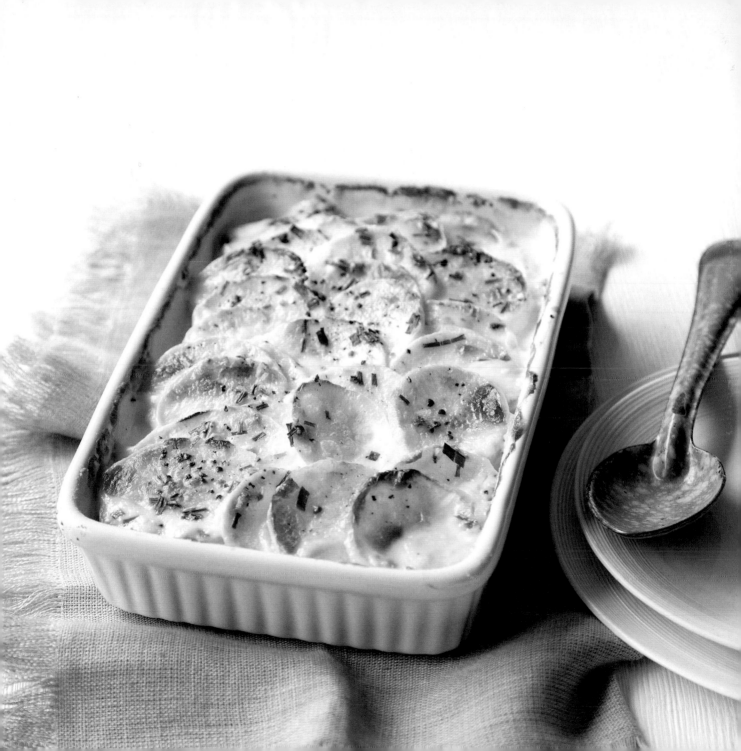

Pumpkin and Swede Mash

This velvety purée is the ideal accompaniment to any particularly juicy dish. Try it with Field Mushrooms with Blue Cheese Custard (see p.46) or, if you're feeding a crowd, Provençal Tian (see p.89). The mash freezes well for future convenience.

500 g/1¼ lb pumpkin,
    trimmed weight, de-seeded,
    peeled and cubed
500 g/1¼ lb swede, trimmed weight,
    peeled and cubed
250 ml/8 fl oz water
2 tbsp whipping cream
Whole nutmeg, for grating
Sea salt and freshly ground
    black pepper

Serves 6

Place the pumpkin and swede in a pan and add water to cover and a pinch of salt. Cover, bring to the boil and cook for 20–30 minutes, until very tender and collapsing. Drain thoroughly (the cooking liquid is a delicious stock which you could save or freeze).

Return the vegetables to the pan and place over a low heat to steam off excess moisture for 5 minutes, stirring frequently. Remove the pan from the heat, add the cream and a very generous grinding of nutmeg. Mash to a smooth purée. Season to taste with salt and pepper and serve.

Per serving
Carbs: 6 g protein: 1 g calories: 50 fibre: 2.5 g fat: 2.5 g (saturated fat: 1 g)

Greens in Coconut Milk

Even those who need a little persuasion to eat their greens might find these hard to refuse. Use Savoy cabbage, kale, spring greens or chard. Brussels sprout tops and purple sprouting broccoli also like this treatment.

1 tbsp olive oil

300 g/11 oz greens, trimmed weight, coarsely chopped or torn

2.5 cm/1 inch piece of fresh root ginger, chopped

400 ml/14 fl oz canned coconut milk

1 tsp ground cumin

Sea salt and freshly ground black pepper

Serves 4

Heat a large pan over a medium heat and add the oil. Add greens and ginger, cover and cook, stirring occasionally, for about 2 minutes, until bright green and wilted.

Add the coconut milk and cumin, season with salt and pepper, and cook, uncovered, for 5 minutes, or until the greens are cooked to your liking. Serve hot.

Per serving
Carbs: 5 g protein: 5 g calories: 222 fibre: 1.5 g fat: 20 g (saturated fat: 12 g)

Baby Courgettes
with Mint and Vinegar

When you see baby courgettes for sale, grab them. They are succulent and naturally sweet. If they have flowers attached, so much the better – this means that they are really fresh and you can add the flowers to this recipe, too. Bulk this up into a main course by adding some slices of buffalo mozzarella and a few rocket leaves. The courgettes can also be cooked on a griddle pan – toss them with the oil in a bowl first, then cook on a preheated griddle pan.

600 g/1 lb 5 oz baby courgettes

2 tbsp olive oil

4 tsp white wine vinegar

A handful of fresh mint leaves,
    coarsely chopped

Salt and freshly ground black pepper

Serves 4

If the courgettes really are young, there's no need to trim them, unless there is a withered flower on one end. If they are larger, trim both ends. Slice in half lengthways.

Heat the oil in a large, non-stick frying pan over a low heat and gently cook the courgettes until well coloured on each side, then remove to a plate. You may have to do this in batches. As each batch comes out of the pan, sprinkle with a little vinegar and season with salt and pepper while still warm. Leave the courgettes to cool completely.

Sprinkle the chopped mint over them and finish with extra pepper.

Per serving
Carbs: 2.5 g protein: 2.6 g calories: 76 fibre: 1.5 g fat: 6 g (saturated fat: 1 g)

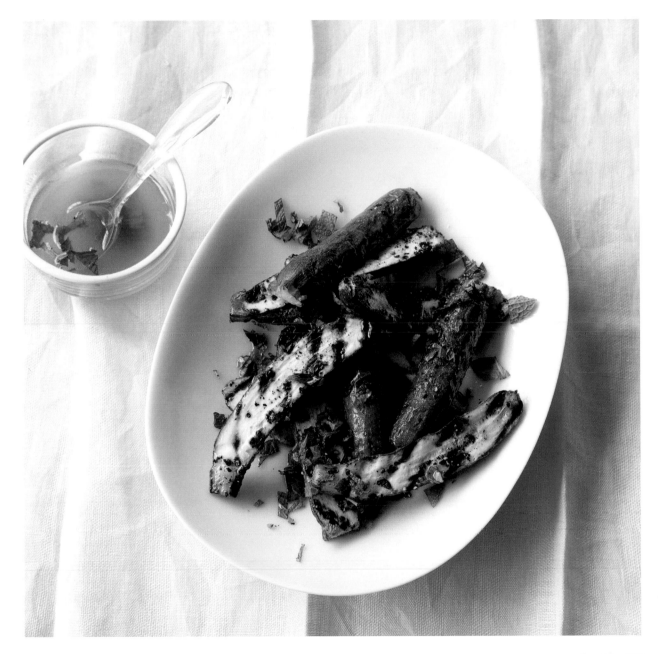

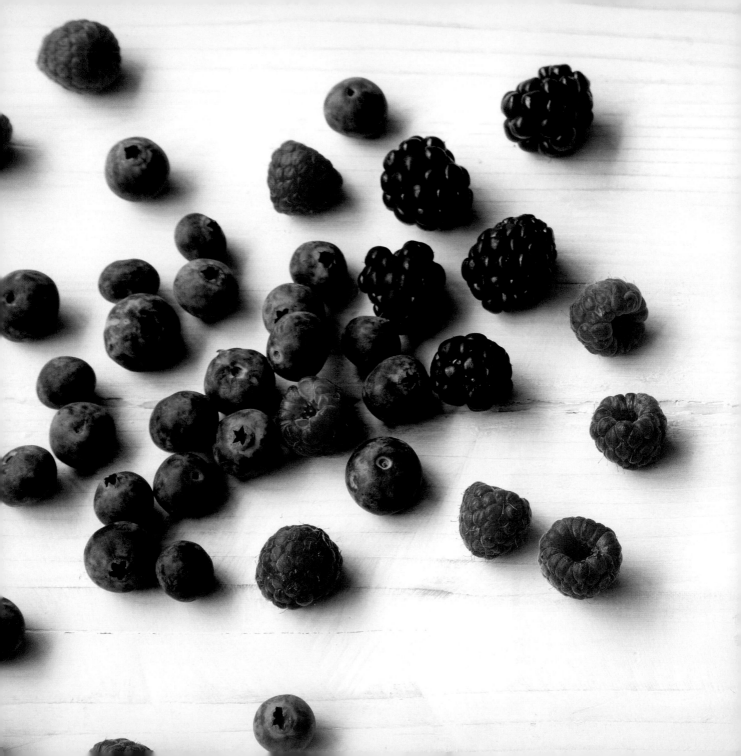

08: SWEET THINGS

Got a sweet tooth? Satiate it here. You needn't deny yourself an indulgent dessert from time to time, with these gratifying sugar-free treats.

Berry Gratin

To enjoy this at its absolute best, a powerful grill is the key, so that the berries are quickly heated to the point of nearly bursting – then they collapse on the tongue.

400 g/14 oz mixed berries,
    especially blackberries,
    raspberries, blueberries
4 tbsp sweetener
150 g/5 oz cream cheese
5 tbsp whipping cream
Juice of ½ a lemon
Coarsely grated rind of 1 lemon

Serves 6

Preheat the grill to its highest setting. Place the berries in a gratin dish and toss 1 tbsp of the sweetener through them.

Beat together the cream cheese, cream, the remaining sweetener and the lemon juice in a bowl. Spoon the mixture over the berries in an even layer, covering most of the surface but leaving a border of berries around the edge. Sprinkle the lemon rind over the top.

Grill for about 5 minutes, or until the topping is patched with gold and the berries are swollen. Serve immediately.

Per serving
Carbs: 4 g protein: 2 g calories: 174 fibre: 2 g fat: 17 g (saturated fat: 10 g)

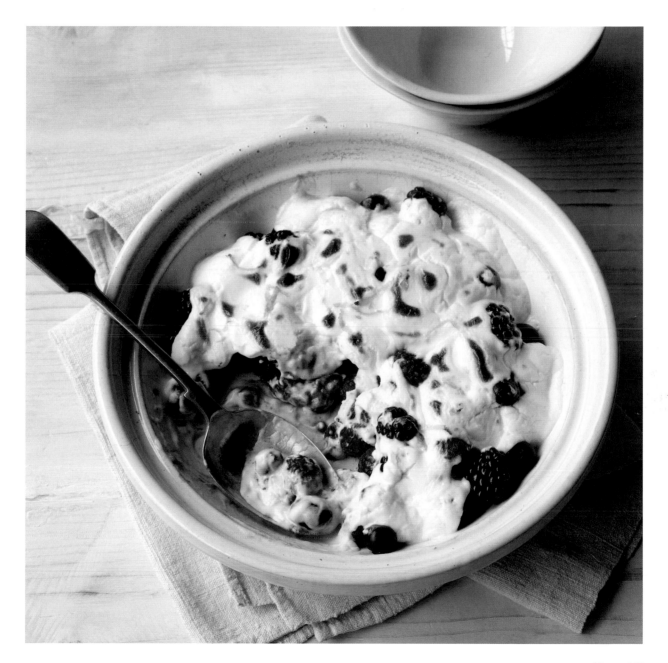

Chocolate Marzipan Cheesecake

A very indulgent cheesecake with a knock-out chocolate flavour and silky texture, perched on a marzipan base.

For the base
100 g/3½ oz ground almonds
50 g/2 oz butter, melted
2 tbsp sweetener
½ tsp almond extract
Good pinch of salt

For the topping
350 g/12 oz cream cheese
150 g/5 oz mascarpone cheese
6 tbsp sweetener
2 organic eggs
150 g/5 oz dark diabetic chocolate, melted
Fresh raspberries, shaved diabetic chocolate, and cocoa powder, to garnish (optional)

Serves 10

Preheat the oven to 150°C/300°F/Gas Mark 2. Put all the ingredients for the base in a bowl and stir to form a thick paste. Press firmly and evenly into the base of a 25 cm/8 inch loose-based cake tin. Chill while you prepare the topping.

Beat together the two cheeses in a bowl with an electric whisk or process in a food processor. Beat in the sweetener and eggs and, finally, the chocolate, beating until smooth. Pour the mixture into the cake tin and bake for 30–40 minutes, until set but still slightly wobbly in the middle.

Leave to cool in the tin (it will set further as it cools). When completely cold, chill in the refrigerator for 3 hours or overnight.

Per serving (ungarnished)
Carbs: 6 g protein: 7 g calories: 402 fibre: 1 g fat: 39 g (saturated fat: 21 g)

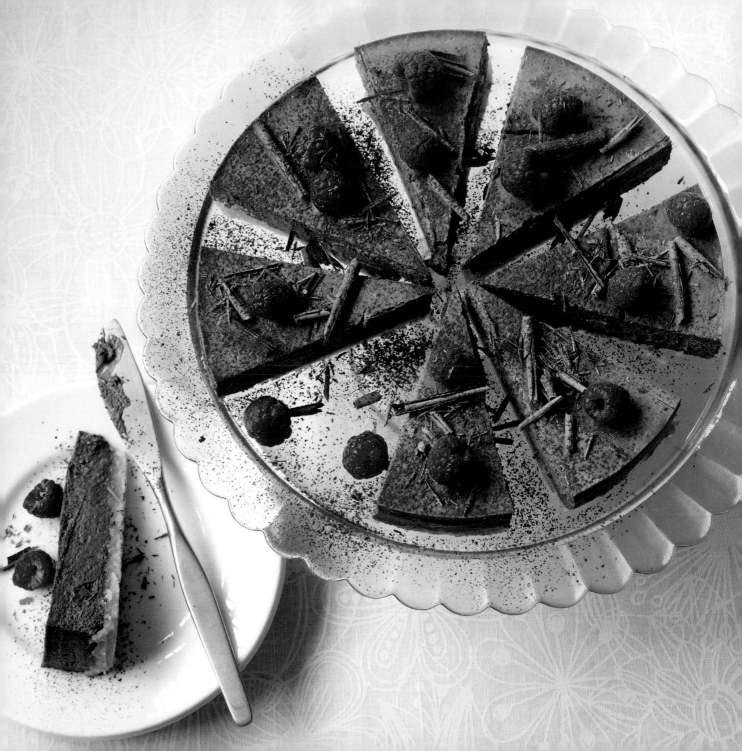

Coconut Ice Cream

This has to be the simplest ice cream ever. Remember to remove it from the freezer at least 30 minutes before serving, or longer. When stirred, you get a floppy, whipped texture just like soft ice cream from an ice cream vendor. Try it with a spoonful of Raspberry Purée (see p.165) drizzled over it. Yum! Yum!

400 ml/14 fl oz can coconut milk
200 ml/7 fl oz double cream
6 tbsp sweetener

Serves 8

Beat all the ingredients together until thoroughly combined. Chill in the refrigerator, then place in an ice-cream maker and follow the manufacturer's instructions.

To freeze the ice cream manually, pour the chilled mixture into a large, shallow plastic container. Cover with a lid and place in the coldest part of the freezer for 1–1½ hours. Remove the container from the freezer and stir the mixture vigorously or beat with an electric mixer, incorporating the ice crystals that will have formed around the edge into the rest of the slush. Cover the container again and return it to the freezer. Repeat this twice more every 2 hours, or until the ice cream is thick throughout. Freeze until ready to serve, then leave at room temperature for at least 30 minutes. Stir before serving.

Per serving
Carbs: 2.5 g protein: 2 g calories: 214 fibre: 0 g fat: 22 g (saturated fat: 15 g)

Coffee Ice Cream

This is a traditional custard-based ice cream. Once you taste the coffee-flavoured custard, you may decide not to freeze it at all and simply devour it as a dessert – it's virtually irresistible.

300 ml/½ pint whipping cream

3 organic egg yolks

3 tbsp sweetener

1 tbsp instant coffee powder

Serves 4

Pour the cream into a pan and gradually bring to just below boiling point over a low to medium heat.

Meanwhile, whisk together the egg yolks, sweetener and instant coffee powder in a jug. The coffee may not immediately dissolve, but don't worry, it soon will.

When the cream just starts to bubble around the edges, remove from the heat and gradually pour it over the egg mixture, whisking constantly. Pour the mixture back into the pan and place it over a low heat. Continue whisking until the mixture becomes thick and coats the back of the spoon.

Pour the mixture back into the rinsed-out jug. Cover with clingfilm and pierce the top so that the steam can escape. Cool, then chill in the refrigerator.

Pour into an ice-cream maker and follow the manufacturer's instructions. Alternatively, follow the instructions for manual ice-cream making, as for Coconut Ice Cream (see p.146).

Per serving
Carbs: 2 g protein: 4 g calories: 331 fibre: 0 g fat: 34 g (saturated fat: 20 g)

Lemon Custard Macaroon Tart

Dried coconut makes a perfect, golden, sweet and crispy tart base.

165 g/5½ oz desiccated coconut

3 organic eggs: 2 separated,
    plus 1 yolk

7 tbsp sweetener

Butter, for greasing

150 ml/5 fl oz double cream

Finely grated zest of 2 lemons

Juice of 1 lemon

Raspberries, to garnish (optional)

Serves 8

Preheat oven to 180°C/350°F/Gas Mark 4. Combine the coconut, 2 egg whites and 3 tbsp of the sweetener in a bowl. Blend until well mixed and sticky. Generously grease a 20 cm/8 inch loose-based, non-stick fluted tart tin and press the coconut mixture firmly into the base and up the sides. Alternatively, use small individual tart tins or a non-stick muffin tin. Place on a baking sheet and bake for 5 minutes.

To make the filling, beat together the 3 egg yolks, the remaining sweetener, the cream, lemon zest and juice. Remove the tart case from the oven and pour in the filling. Return to the oven for 15 minutes, until patched with gold.

Leave to cool completely before removing from the tin, using the end of a small knife to loosen the edges.

Per serving (ungarnished)
Carbs: 2 g protein: 2 g calories: 226 fibre: 3 g fat: 24 g (saturated fat: 17 g)

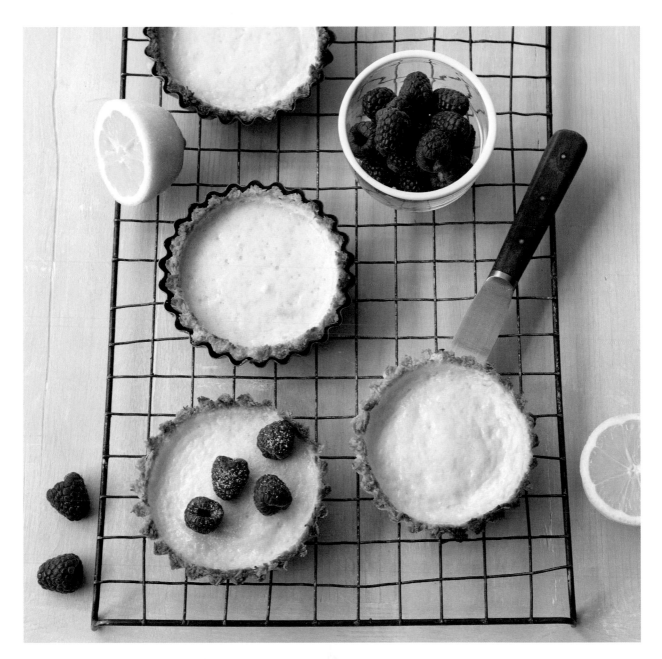

Zabaglione

There's a fair amount of continuous whisking involved in zabaglione, so it's most comfortably made for just two people. It should also be eaten immediately – warm, boozy and frothy. It's a wonderful spontaneous dessert. Enjoy on its own or with 1–2 spoonfuls of Raspberry Purée (see p.165) stirred through.

4 organic egg yolks

2 tbsp sweetener

4 tbsp Marsala wine
   or Madeira or sherry

Serves 2

Pour about a 2.5 cm/1 inch depth of water into a pan, over which you can set a small heatproof glass bowl. Bring to the boil.

Meanwhile, beat all the ingredients together in the heatproof bowl until evenly combined. Reduce the boiling water to a simmer and set the bowl over it. Whisk constantly for 4–5 minutes, until the mixture has nearly trebled in volume and begins to hold its shape. Serve immediately.

Per serving
Carbs: 4 g protein: 37 g calories: 450 fibre: 0 g fat: 27 g (saturated fat: 8 g)

Cardamom Cake

Cardamom has the ability to make things taste sweeter, so I knew it would be ideal in a low-carb recipe. A sliver of this light sponge cake is perfect with coffee or afternoon tea.

Butter, for greasing

75 g/3 oz soy flour

50 g/2 oz ground almonds

1 tsp baking powder

1 tsp cardamom seeds,
    out of the pod, crushed

5 tbsp sweetener

2 organic eggs

3 tbsp reduced-fat crème fraîche
    or sour cream

3 tbsp sunflower oil

1 tbsp vanilla extract

Generous pinch of salt

Serves 8

Preheat the oven to 180°C/350°F/Gas Mark 4. Grease a 20 cm/8 inch cake tin and line the base with baking parchment.

Stir together the flour, ground almonds, baking powder and cardamom seeds in a small bowl.

In a separate bowl, using an electric whisk or by hand, beat together the sweetener, eggs, crème fraîche or sour cream, oil, vanilla and salt. Stir the dry ingredients into the wet, combining thoroughly, but do not over-work. Pour into the prepared tin and bake for 20 minutes, until golden and set. Rest for 5 minutes, then turn out onto a wire rack to cool.

Per serving
Carbs: 3 g protein: 7.5 g calories: 140 fibre: 5 g fat: 11 g (saturated fat: 1.8 g)

Cream Cheese and Macadamia Nut Brownies

High-impact, real brownies, studded with rich macadamias and pockets of baked cream cheese.

150 g/5 oz dark diabetic chocolate, chopped

100 g/3½ oz butter

3 organic eggs

5 tbsp sweetener

1 tsp vanilla extract

75 g/3 oz soy flour

1 tsp baking powder

Pinch of salt

100 g/3½ oz unsalted macadamia nuts, coarsely chopped

75 g/3 oz chilled cream cheese, cut into small cubes

Makes 12

Preheat the oven to 180°C/350°F/Gas Mark 4. Line a small rectangular cake tin or ovenproof dish with baking parchment.

Melt the chocolate and butter together in a heatproof bowl set over a pan of simmering water. Alternatively, melt in the microwave. Stir until smooth, then leave to cool slightly.

Beat together the eggs, sweetener and vanilla in a large bowl. Add the chocolate mixture and combine thoroughly. Sift the flour, baking powder and salt over the mixture, add the nuts and stir until just mixed.

Pour into the prepared tin or dish and smooth the surface. Dot with the cream cheese. Bake for 30–40 minutes, until firm. Cool, then cut into 12 squares.

Per serving
Carbs: 7 g protein: 6 g calories: 257 fibre: 1 g fat: 23 g (saturated fat: 10 g)

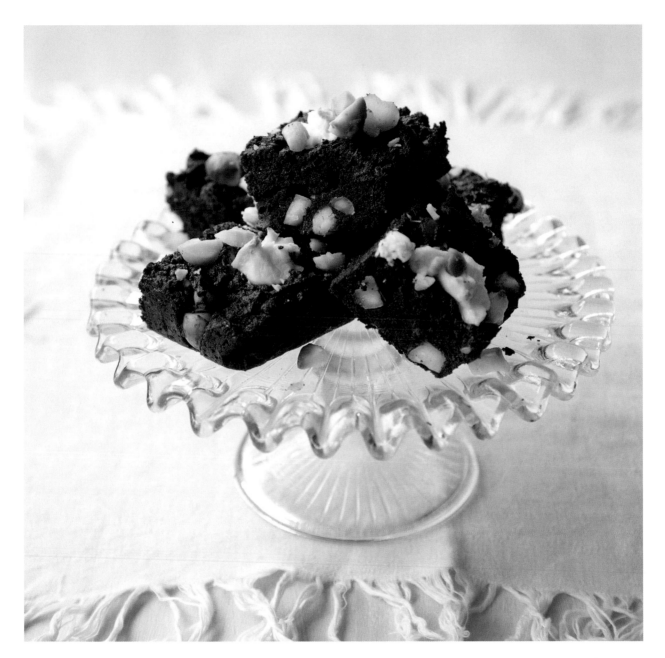

Rose and Raspberry Pudding

The delicate taste of rosewater is the surprise element in this raspberry-flecked custard. I like to use frozen raspberries, because they ooze their magenta juices as they defrost in the cooling pudding. Rosewater varies greatly in strength, so start with a smaller amount and increase if desired.

150 g/5 oz fresh or frozen raspberries

6 organic egg yolks

4 tbsp sweetener

1–3 tbsp rosewater, to taste

600 ml/1 pint double cream

1 vanilla pod

Serves 6

Divide the raspberries among 6 individual wine glasses or small bowls and set aside.

Place the egg yolks, sweetener and rosewater in a large bowl and hand-whisk until smooth.

Pour the cream into a pan. Slit the vanilla pod lengthways and scrape out the seeds into the cream, then place the pod in the cream and bring gently to just below simmering point – it should just start to bubble around the edges. Remove the pod and gradually pour the hot cream over the egg mixture, whisking constantly. Pour the mixture back into the pan and whisk over a low heat until thick. Pour the custard into the prepared glasses or bowls. Leave to cool, then chill.

Per serving
Carbs: 3 g protein: 5 g calories: 563 fibre: 0.6 g fat: 60 g (saturated fat: 35 g)

Chocolate Truffles

These delectable truffles are the perfect little mouthful to round off dinner with a black coffee or brandy. If you use a high-quality diabetic chocolate, no-one will believe they're sugar-free. Wearing latex or plastic gloves makes rolling the truffle mixture easier. You will probably get through several changes of gloves.

250 g/8 oz dark diabetic chocolate, broken into pieces
50 g/2 oz butter
175 ml/6 fl oz double cream
6 tbsp unsweetened pure cocoa powder

Makes 35

Place the chocolate in a food processor and pulse until very finely chopped.

Place the butter and cream in a pan and heat gently just until the butter has melted. Remove the pan from the heat and stir in the chocolate. Continue to stir until smooth. If the mixture is too hot, it may separate; if this happens, add more cream.

Pour the mixture into a flat dish that will fit in the refrigerator. Leave to cool, then chill until firm.

Place the cocoa powder in a bowl. Remove the truffle mixture from the refrigerator. Scrape up cherry-size lumps of mixture and roll into smooth balls. Drop into the bowl of cocoa. Prepare a few at a time, shake them around in the cocoa to coat evenly, then remove to a plate. Continue until you have used up all of the truffle mixture.

Chill the truffles until ready to use.

Per serving
Carbs: 3 g protein: 0.9 g calories: 71 fibre: 0 g fat: 6.3 g (saturated fat: 3.9 g)

Pistachio Meringues

These are quite different from traditional meringues, but quite wonderful in their own right. They are feather-light and literally melt in the mouth while being crunchy at the same time. Pistachios make them extra special, but you could use hazelnuts or almonds instead.

100 g/3½ oz shelled pistachios (weight without shell)
2 egg whites
Pinch of cream of tartar
6 tbsp sweetener

Makes 8

Preheat oven to 120°C/250°F/Gas Mark ½. Line a baking sheet with baking parchment.

Grind the pistachios to a powder in a food processor or chop as finely as possible by hand. Beat the egg whites with cream of tartar in a grease-free bowl until stiff. Beat in the sweetener. Gently fold in the ground pistachios, keeping the mixture light and airy.

Spoon little mounds of the mixture on to the baking sheet. Bake for 30–40 minutes, until crisp and golden.

Per serving
Carbs: 1 g protein: 3 g calories: 78 fibre: 0.8 g fat: 7 g (saturated fat: 1 g)

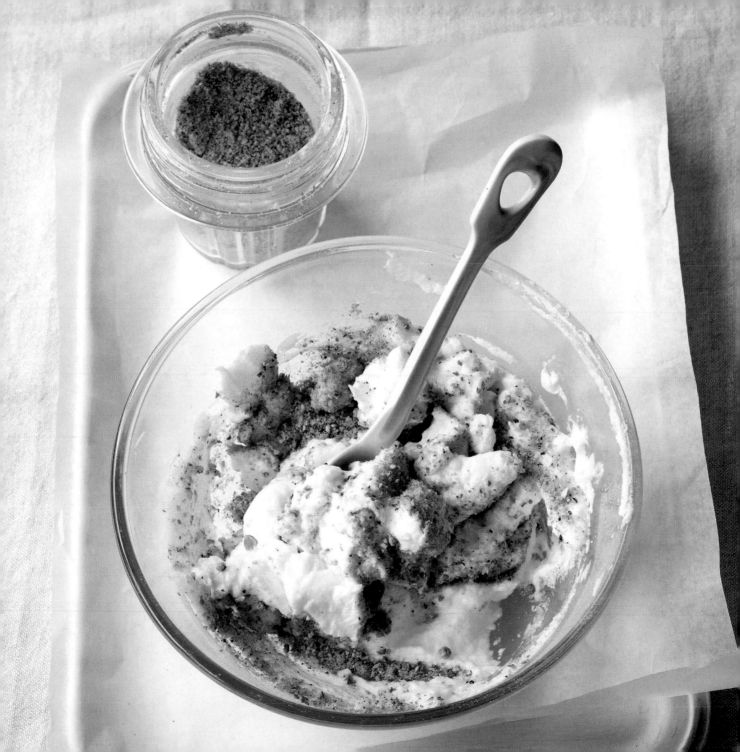

Rhubarb Fool

Low-carb sweeteners taste particularly authentic with acidic foods, so rhubarb is a perfect foil and is itself low-carb. Ginger, also a great partner to rhubarb, makes this quintessentially English dessert complete.

400 g/14 oz rhubarb, trimmed
    and cut into 1 cm/½ inch pieces
3 tbsp water
2 tsp finely grated fresh root ginger
Pinch of salt
4 tbsp sweetener
300 ml/½ pint double cream

Serves 6

Place the rhubarb, water, ginger and salt in a non-reactive pan (that is, not aluminium), cover and bring to the boil. Reduce the heat to a low simmer and stew for about 15 minutes, until the rhubarb has collapsed. Strain off some of the liquid through a non-aluminium sieve, then place in a ceramic or glass bowl and leave to cool.

When cool, add sweetener to taste. Whip the cream until it holds its shape, then fold in the rhubarb, so it streaks through the cream in pink ripples, but isn't completely homogenous. Spoon into four glasses and chill for at least 30 minutes before serving.

Per serving
Carbs: 2 g protein: 2 g calories: 380 fibre: 1.5 g fat: 40 g (saturated fat: 25 g)

Eton Mess

Here's a rather nuttier version of the English summertime classic, made with Pistachio Meringues (see p.156). A touch of rosewater enhances the sweetness. Use strawberries instead of raspberries if that's what's available.

1 quantity Pistachio Meringues
(see p.156)
250 ml/8 fl oz double cream
150 g/5 oz raspberries
1 tsp rosewater

Serves 6

Whisk the cream until it holds its shape, but do not over-whisk.

Place the meringues in a large bowl and break up slightly. Add the raspberries and cream and fold through, trying not to flatten the meringues. Gently fold the rosewater through the mixture. Serve immediately.

Per serving
Carbs: 3.3 g protein: 6 g calories: 484 fibre: 2.5 g fat: 49 g (saturated fat: 26 g)

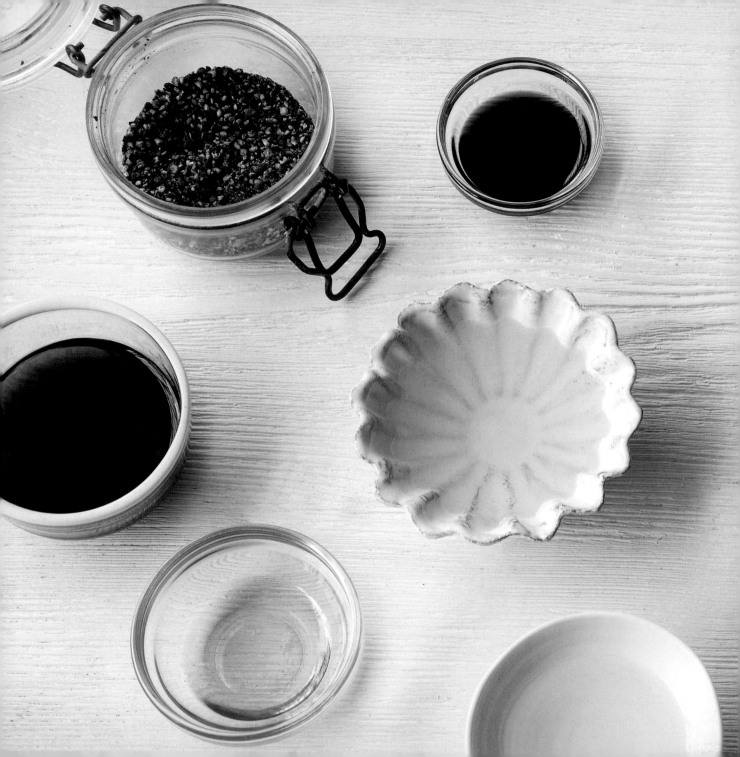

09:
FLAVOUR
ESSENTIALS

A few basics, with dressings and sauces specially designed to inject flavour, colour and texture into just about anything that fails to excite. With these essential recipes in your repertoire, you can create your own low-carb dishes.

Vegetable Stock

Homemade vegetable stock will make your soups and stews taste better than a powder or cube, and will always be guaranteed virtually carb-less, if you follow my guidelines below. Alas, life doesn't always allow us the luxury of time to make it (although it only takes about half an hour) – but if you can make a large batch, freeze it in 250 ml/½ pint portions in zip-seal plastic bags. Also, save the water left from steaming and blanching vegetables and freeze the same way.

Vegetables (see list below)
Water (quantity to suit)
Sea salt
Peppercorns

GOOD in stock:
Spring onions
Garlic
Celery and celery leaves
Parsley and parsley stems
Leeks and well-washed leek greens
Broccoli and broccoli stems
Courgettes
Fennel and fennel tops
Turnips
Woody herbs such as rosemary
    and thyme
Bay leaves

AVOID in stock:
Cabbage, spring greens,
    collard greens, kale
Cauliflower
Brussels sprouts
Potatoes and any other
    starchy vegetables

Fill half a large pot with items from the "Good" list. Add enough water to cover the vegetables. Add sea salt to taste and a small handful of peppercorns. Bring to the boil and simmer for 20–30 minutes, then strain. Use immediately, or cool and keep chilled for up to 3 days. Alternatively, freeze as described above.

Per 300 ml/½ pint serving
Carbs: 0.8 g protein: 2 g calories: 16 fibre: 0 g fat: 0.2 g (saturated fat: 0 g)

Paneer

This homemade curd cheese is a staple of the Indian diet. It's high in protein and has a wonderful creamy yet chewy texture. It is sold in some supermarkets and Asian groceries, but when you discover how easy it is to make yourself, you'll be a convert – all you have to do is separate milk into curds and whey. The homemade stuff is also infinitely lighter and creamier.

3.5 litres/6 pints full-cream milk
100 ml/3½ fl oz strained freshly
    squeezed lemon juice

Makes about 300 g/10½ oz

Bring the milk to the boil in a large pan. As soon as it starts to rise up the sides of the pan, turn off the heat. Stir in the lemon juice. Cover the pan and leave to stand for 10 minutes.

Drain the curds in a colander lined with muslin or a clean tea towel. When cool enough to handle, squeeze out the excess moisture and leave to cool and drain further, then chill.

Paneer can be used once it has cooled, although it will have a very crumbly texture. It will harden enough to slice within 1 hour in the refrigerator, and will harden further the longer it's chilled.

Per 75 g/3 oz serving
Carbs: 2 g protein: 9 g calories: 76 fibre: 0 g fat: 3 g (saturated fat: 1.5 g)

Blender Hollandaise

It's just about the most sinful sauce around – all that butter – but if you're sticking to your low-carb diet, a little of this won't blow it for you. This foolproof version has a particular affinity with steamed asparagus, and it's an essential part of Eggs Florentine (see p.28).

3 organic egg yolks
2 tbsp water
1 tbsp fresh lemon juice
150 g/5 oz lightly salted butter,
diced

Serves 4

Place the egg yolks, water and lemon juice in a blender.

Place the butter in a pan over a very low heat. As soon as it has melted, remove from the heat but do not let it cool.

Switch on the blender, then gradually pour the hot melted butter through the hole in the lid to produce a thick and creamy emulsion.

If the sauce needs to be kept for a short time before use, it can be poured into a heatproof bowl, covered and set over a pan of hot water (not actively simmering) to keep warm. It will solidify if stored in the refrigerator, but reheats successfully in a microwave.

Per serving
Carbs: 0.2 g protein: 2 g calories: 325 fibre: 0 g fat: 35 g (saturated fat: 20 g)

Pesto

There's plenty else to enjoy pesto with other than traditional pasta: look out for the amazing range of carb-free and low-carb pasta, noodles and rice available online and in specialty shops. Try it stirred through spaghetti squash (see p.80 for cooking instructions), as a dressing for boiled turnips, pumpkin or cauliflower, or as an uplifting companion for crunchy vegetables such as celery (see Celery with Pesto, p.111).

Large bunch of fresh basil,
 stems and leaves, torn
100 g/3½ oz pine nuts
2 garlic cloves
50 g/2 oz freshly grated
 Parmesan cheese
Salt
6 tbsp olive oil

Serves 4

Place the basil, pine nuts, garlic, Parmesan and a pinch of salt in a food processor. Process until finely chopped, then, with the motor running, gradually add the oil. Taste for seasoning and add more salt if necessary. Store in an airtight container in the refrigerator for up to 3 days, or freeze.

Per serving
Carbs: 1 g protein: 9 g calories: 382 fibre: 0.5 g fat: 38 g (saturated fat: 6 g)

Raspberry Purée

This pink purée poses as a sweet sauce, flavouring (see Zabaglione, p.150) or as a low-carb jam substitute (see Cottage Cheese Pancakes, p.31).

75 g/3 oz raspberries
1½ tbsp water
1 tbsp sweetener

Makes about 125 ml/4 fl oz

Serves 4

Place all the ingredients in a blender and process until smooth. Pass through a sieve. The purée can be stored in the refrigerator for up to 3 days, or can be frozen.

Per serving
Carbs: 0.9 g protein: 0.3 g calories: 5 fibre: 0.5 g fat: 0.1 g (saturated fat: 0 g)

Sweet Chilli Sauce

This basic sauce is a perfect balance of sweet, sour, salty and hot – the principle behind the moreish flavour of South-East Asian food.

2 tbsp fresh lime juice
2 tbsp light soy sauce
2 tbsp sweetener
2 small hot red chillies,
  finely chopped
1 small garlic clove, crushed
  or finely grated

Serves 4

Combine all the ingredients. The heat will increase the longer it stands.

Per serving
Carbs: 0 g protein: 0.2 g calories: 3 fibre: 0.6 g fat: 0 g (saturated fat: 0 g)

Coconut Chilli Sauce

This is a fantastic marinade for tofu or a quick way to liven up steamed vegetables. It's also delicious with hard-boiled eggs. It uses ready-made chilli sauce so check the label to make sure it's a low-carb version with no sugar or modified starch.

5 tbsp coconut milk or coconut cream
2 tsp low-carb chilli sauce or several
  shakes of Tabasco sauce
2 tsp light soy sauce
1 tsp fresh lime juice
1 tsp sweetener

Serves 4

Mix all ingredients together and serve. The sauce may solidify if it is kept in the refrigerator; return to room temperature before use.

Per serving
Carbs: 1 g protein: 0.6 g calories: 35 fibre: 0 g fat: 3.2 g (saturated fat: 2 g)

Basic Vinaigrette

A heavy mortar and pestle is one of the most useful tools in the kitchen. This is how you will get the very best flavour out of garlic as the base for any vinaigrette or sauce.

1 garlic clove

1 tsp coarse sea salt

2 tbsp white wine vinegar

1 tsp dry mustard

½ tsp mixed dried herbs
    or Herbes de Provence

Freshly ground black pepper

3 tbsp extra virgin olive oil

Serves 4

Using a mortar and pestle, pound the garlic with the salt until a smooth paste forms. Using the pestle, work in the vinegar, mustard and herbs, and season to taste with pepper. Gradually whisk in the olive oil.

Per serving
Carbs: 0 g protein: 0 g calories: 75 fibre: 0 g fat: 8 g (saturated fat: 1 g)

Cheese Sauce

This rich sauce will make just about anything more exciting – try it spooned over a plate of steamed broccoli and courgettes with hard-boiled eggs or smoked tofu.

120 ml/4 fl oz Vegetable Stock
    (see p.162)

100 g/3½ oz cream cheese

50 g/2 oz grated Gruyère, Cheddar,
    or other mature, tangy cheese

½ tsp dry mustard (optional)

½ tsp fresh or dried thyme leaves
    (optional)

Serves 4

Bring the stock to the boil in a frying pan. Add the cream cheese, breaking it up with a whisk. Whisk until smooth and melted.

Add the grated cheese, mustard and thyme, if using, and whisk until the cheese has melted and the sauce is thick. Remove from the heat and serve immediately.

Per serving
Carbs: 0.4 g protein: 5 g calories: 165 fibre: 0 g fat: 16 g (saturated fat: 10 g)

Italian Blue Cheese Dressing

The true, original blue cheese dressing – before it came out of labelled bottles – for all kinds of salads. Make sure the cheese is at room temperature before you start.

100 g/3½ oz Gorgonzola cremosa,
    Dolcelatte, or other soft blue
    cheese
1 tbsp white wine vinegar
2 tbsp extra-virgin olive oil
Sea salt and freshly ground
    black pepper

Makes about 100 ml/3½ fl oz

Serves 4

Remove and discard any rind from the cheese. Place the cheese in a bowl and break it up slightly with a fork, then beat in the vinegar. Beat in the oil with a pinch of salt and pepper. This dressing will keep in the refrigerator for up to 3 days.

Per serving
Carbs: 0.2 g protein: 6 g calories: 152 fibre: 0 g fat: 14 g (saturated fat: 6.5 g)

Sesame Vinaigrette

A light salad dressing with an Asian twist, this is also a good tofu marinade.

1 tbsp sesame seeds
2 tbsp dark soy sauce
2 tbsp rice vinegar
2 tbsp sesame oil

Makes about 100 ml/3½ fl oz

Serves 4

Place the sesame seeds in a small, dry frying pan and set over a medium heat. Cook, shaking the pan and stirring frequently, until the seeds are popping and golden. Transfer to a bowl and leave to cool.

Beat the remaining ingredients into the toasted sesame seeds. Use immediately, while the seeds are still crunchy.

Per serving
Carbs: 0.6 g protein: 1 g calories: 75 fibre: 0.3 g fat: 8 g (saturated fat: 1 g)

Sesame Mayo

Here's an example of how the magical combination of three ingredients adds up to more than the sum of its parts. This versatile sauce/dressing/dip just goes with everything!

3 tbsp sesame seeds
120 ml/4 fl oz mayonnaise
1½ tbsp dark soy sauce

Makes 120 ml/4 fl oz

Serves 4

Place the sesame seeds in a small, dry frying pan and set over a medium heat. Cook, shaking the pan and stirring frequently, until the seeds are popping and golden. Transfer to a bowl and leave to cool.

Add the mayonnaise and soy sauce and combine thoroughly. The sauce is best eaten on the day you make it, as the sesame seeds tend to become soggy after a while.

Per serving
Carbs: 0.3 g protein: 1 g calories: 137 fibre: 0.3 g fat: 15 g (saturated fat: 2 g)

Satay Sauce

This sauce or dressing provides a speedy flavour injection. Make a quick *Gado-Gado* salad with hard-boiled eggs, lettuce or shredded cabbage, bean sprouts, a few pepper strips and sliced spring onion, then smother it in this dressing.

3 tbsp crunchy natural peanut butter
2 tbsp boiling water
2 tsp low-carb store-bought
    chilli sauce
1 tsp fresh lime juice
1 tsp sweetener
Soy sauce, to taste (optional)

Makes about 100 ml/3½ fl oz

Place the peanut butter in a small bowl and pour over the boiling water. Beat with a fork until thoroughly combined. Beat in the remaining ingredients and taste for seasoning. Beat in a little soy sauce for extra saltiness, if desired.

Per serving
Carbs: 1 g protein: 2 g calories: 50 fibre: 0.5 g fat: 4 g (saturated fat: 1 g)

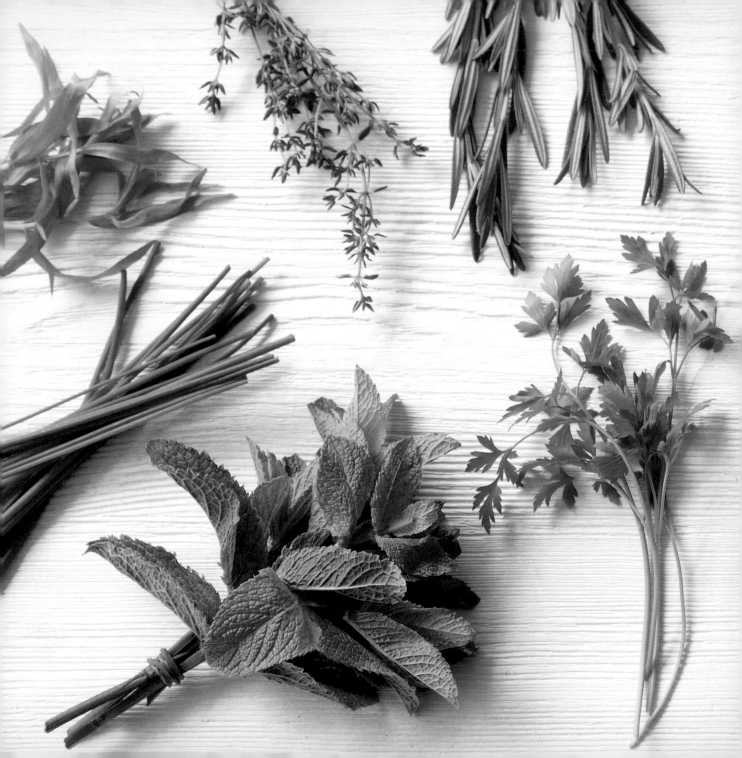

MENU
IDEAS

BRUNCH BUFFET
Japanese Omelette, *p.25*
Blueberry Almond Griddle Cakes, *p.18*
Almond Muffins with Butter, *p.33*
Melon Berry Power Smoothie, *p.21*
Black Coffee

MEDITERRANEAN MEZE
Olive Raisins, *p.100*
Halloumi-Stuffed Peppers, *p.48*
Smoked Aubergine Purée, *p.125*
Citrus Chilli Labneh Platter, *p.122*
Fruity Red Wine

AL FRESCO LUNCH
Spanish Tortilla with Courgette and Manchego, *p.66*
Green Bean and Roasted Pepper Parcels, *p.116*
A Crisp Green Salad Served with Italian Blue Cheese Dressing, *p.168*
Chilled Prosecco

PICNIC
Tunisian Spiced Torte, *p.84*
Marinated Crudité Salad, *p.110*
Cream Cheese and Macadamia Nut Brownies, *p.152*
Iced Tea with Lemon and Sweetener

LUNCH BUFFET
Field Mushrooms with Blue Cheese Custard, *p.46*
Provençal Tian, *p.89*
Avocado and Lemon Salad, *p.128*
Chocolate Marzipan Cheesecake, *p.144*

EASY ASIAN BUFFET
Tofu, Mint and Palm Heart Salad, *p.60*
Vietnamese Asparagus Pancakes, *p.70*
Gado-Gado Salad, see Satay Sauce intro, *p.169*
Coconut Ice Cream, *p.146*

LUNCH BOX
Spanish Tortilla with Courgettes and Manchego, *p.66*
Spicy Tofu Biltong, *p.106*
Almond Muffin, *p.33*

WARMING WINTER LUNCH
Curried Celeriac Soup with Coriander Oil, *p.56*
Warm Salad of Aubergine and Melting Camembert, *p.75*
Zabaglione, *p.150*

SPEEDY AFTER-WORK DINNER 1
Chinese-Spice Tofu and Baby Leaf Salad, *p.59*
Egg Foo Yung, *p.86*

SPEEDY AFTER-WORK DINNER 2
Egg Flower Soup, *p.40*
Warm Exotic Mushroom Salad, *p.62*

THAI FEAST
Cucumber and Tofu Satay, *p.118*
Fragrant Coconut Broth, *p.36*
Thai Hot and Sour Salad with Crispy Tofu, *p.78*
Coconut Ice Cream, *p.146*
Jasmine Tea

INDIAN FEAST
Spiced Charred Aubergines, *p.51*
Paneer and Herb Fritters, *p.92*
Pumpkin and Egg Curry, *p.94*
Rose and Raspberry Pudding, *p.154*
Low-Carb Beer

COCKTAIL BASH
Chilli-Crust Brazil Nuts, *p.100*
Saffron Aïoli with Quail's Eggs and Asparagus, *p.120*
Aubergine and Smoked Cheese Involtini, *p.114*
Cucumber with Pink Pickled Ginger, *p.117*
Chocolate Truffles, *p.155*
Vodka Martinis

FOUR-COURSE RED-CARPET DINNER
Tricolore Skewers (with Champagne), *p.117*
Red Pepper and Goat's Cheese Timbales, *p.45*
Warm Poached Egg Salad with Tarragon Vinaigrette, *p.64*
Chilled White Burgundy
Individual Berry Gratins, *p.142*
Cognac and Black Coffee

INDEX